LRC Radbrook

MENTAL HEALTH LAW

A PRACTICAL GUIDE

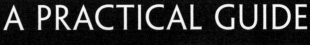 KT-514-549

Basant K. Puri MA, PhD, MB, BChir, BSc (Hons) MathSci, MRCPsych, DipStat, MMath
Professor of Imaging Psychiatry, MRI Unit, Imaging Sciences Department, Faculty of Medicine, MRC Clinical Sciences Centre, Hammersmith Hospital and Imperial College, London; and Honorary Consultant in Imaging, Department of Radiology, Hammersmith Hospitals NHS Trust, London, UK

Robert A. Brown MA Applied Social Studies
Course Director for the Approved Social Workers course in South West England, Mental Health Act Commissioner, Visiting Fellow Bournemouth University, Bournemouth, UK

Heather J. McKee MB, ChB, BAO, MRCPsych, LLM
Consultant Psychiatrist, West London Mental Health NHS Trust, London; and Honorary Senior Lecturer, Imperial College School of Medicine, London, UK

Ian H. Treasaden MB, BS, LRCP, MRCS, MRCPsych
Consultant Forensic Psychiatrist and Clinical Director, Three Bridges Medium Secure Unit, West London Mental Health NHS Trust, London; and Honorary Clinical Senior Lecturer in Forensic Psychiatry, Imperial College School of Medicine, London, UK

Hodder Arnold
A MEMBER OF THE HODDER HEADLINE GROUP

First published in Great Britain in 2005 by
Hodder Education, a member of the Hodder Headline Group,
338 Euston Road, London NW1 3BH. Reprinted 2006

http://www.hoddereducation.com

Distributed in the United States of America by
Oxford University Press Inc.,
198 Madison Avenue, New York, NY10016
Oxford is a registered trademark of Oxford University Press

© 2005 Basant K. Puri, Robert A. Brown, Heather J. McKee and Ian H. Treasaden

All rights reserved. Apart from any use permitted under UK copyright law,
this publication may only be reproduced, stored or transmitted, in any form,
or by any means with prior permission in writing of the publishers or in the
case of reprographic production in accordance with the terms of licences
issued by the Copyright Licensing Agency. In the United Kingdom such
licences are issued by the Copyright Licensing Agency: 90 Tottenham Court
Road, London W1T 4LP.

While the advice and information in this book are believed to be true and
accurate at the date of going to press, neither the authors nor the publisher can
accept any legal responsibility or liability for any errors or omissions that may
have been made. In particular (but without limiting the generality of the preceding
disclaimer) while every effort has been made to check the latest developments in
legislation and case law, recent developments may not be reflected here. The reader
is therefore strongly urged to consult the latest court reports, Government websites
and other legal reference material as an up-to-date adjunct to the guidance provided
in this book.

British Library Cataloguing in Publication Data
A catalogue record for this book is available from the British Library

Library of Congress Cataloging-in-Publication Data
A catalog record for this book is available from the Library of Congress

ISBN-10: 0 340 88503 3
ISBN-13: 978 0 340 88503 1

2 3 4 5 6 7 8 9 10

Commissioning Editor: Georgina Bentliff
Project Editor: Heather Smith
Production Controller: Jane Lawrence
Cover Design: Amina Dudhia

Typeset in 9.5 on 12pt New Baskerville by Phoenix Photosetting, Chatham, Kent
Printed and bound in Spain

Hodder Headline's policy is to use papers that are natural, renewable and recyclable products
and made from wood grown in sustainable forests. The logging and manufacturing processes
are expected to conform to the environmental regulations of the country of origin.

What do you think about this book? Or any other Hodder Arnold title?
Please visit our website at www.hoddereducation.com

Contents

Contributors

Christine Dixon MRPharmS
Principal Pharmacist, Epsom General Hospital, Epsom, Surrey, UK

Angela Hassiotis MA, MRCPsych
Senior Lecturer in the Psychiatry of Learning Disabilities, Royal Free and University College Medical School, Department of Mental Health, London, UK

Paul J. Laking MB, ChB, MRCPsych
Consultant Psychiatrist, Suffolk Mental Health Partnerships Trust, Ipswich, UK

Legal advisors

Sections of the manuscript related to mental health law and to criminal law were reviewed by the following advisors, who made suggestions and recommendations to the authors on the basis of their specialist experience and knowledge of current law and legal practice. Their help is much appreciated. The final version of the text is the work of the authors, incorporating those suggestions and recommendations as the authors have judged best:

David Nicolls BA (Hons) Law (Advisor in Criminal Law)
Head of Criminal Department, Levenes Solicitors, London, UK

Helen Kingston BA (Hons) Law (Advisor in the Mental Health Act)
Solicitor, Eversheds Solicitors, Newcastle, UK

Preface

One of the hallmarks of a civilized society is the way in which it caters for those who require help as a result of mental health problems. Mental health legislation has generally developed internationally from that which protected society from people with mental disorder to additionally protecting the health and safety of people with mental disorder. In providing the legal structure within which such people may be compulsorily detained and treated, if necessary against their will, a balance must be struck between, on the one hand, the rights of an individual in a free society and, on the other hand, the need to protect the individual, and society at large, from the adverse effects of mental disorders. This handbook describes the ways in which the Mental Health Act 1983 (England and Wales) achieves these aims.

We are mindful of the fact that historically, the legislators of many other countries have looked to the England and Wales Mental Health Act for guidance when formulating their own mental health legislation. We ourselves hope we have avoided being too parochial by including international comparisons with mental health legislation outside of England and Wales.

This handbook is meant to be a portable and practical guide to the use of the Mental Health Act. We trust it will be of value to psychiatrists (at all stages of their careers), nurses, social workers, general practitioners, police surgeons, accident-and-emergency hospital staff, prison medical officers, psychologists, probation officers, hospital administrators, members of the legal profession, and lay members of tribunals. Others involved in the care of people suffering from mental disorders may also find this book of use.

We thank Dr Paul J. Laking and Dr Angela Hassiotis for contributing the chapters on children's mental health law and people with learning disabilities, respectively. We are grateful to Paul Barber (Consultant with Bevan Ashford) for the case law summaries. We should also like to thank our publishers, Arnold, for their patient nurturing of this handbook since its inception; particular thanks are due to Georgina Bentliff, Heather Smith and Serena Bureau.

HL v THE UNITED KINGDOM, EUROPEAN COURT JUDGMENT, OCTOBER 2004

This is the final stage of the Bournewood case and has major implications for English mental health law. Extracts from the judgment, which was published just as this book was going to press, are reproduced below.

"The applicant was born in 1949 and lives in Surrey. He has suffered from autism since birth. He is unable to speak and his level of understanding is limited. He is frequently agitated and has a history of self-harming behaviour. He lacks the capacity to consent or object to medical treatment. For over 30 years he was cared for in Bournewood Hospital ... He was an inpatient at the Intensive Behavioural Unit (IBU) from 1987. The applicant's responsible medical officer (who had cared for him since 1977) was Dr M … In March 1994 he was discharged on a trial basis to paid carers, Mr and Mrs E, with whom he successfully resided until 22 July 1997 [when] he was at the day centre when he became particularly agitated, hitting himself on the head with his fists and banging his head against the wall. Staff could not contact Mr and Mrs E and got in touch with a local doctor who administered a sedative."

HL remained agitated and on the recommendation of the local authority care services manager with overall responsibility for the applicant, he was taken to the A&E unit at the hospital. He was seen by a psychiatrist and transferred to the IBU. It was recorded that he made no attempt to leave. "Dr P and Dr M considered that the best interests of the applicant required his admission for in-patient treatment".

Dr M considered detention under the 1983 Act but concluded it "was not necessary as the applicant was compliant and did not resist admission". Dr M later confirmed that she would have recommended HL's detention if he had resisted admission. The carers were discouraged from visiting at this point. In a report on August 18 Dr M concluded that HL suffered from a mood disorder as well as autism and that his discharge would be against medical opinion.

On October 29 1997 the Court of Appeal indicated it would decide the appeal in the applicant's favour. HL was then held on Section 5(2) and on October 31 an application for section 3 was made. On November 2 he was seen by his carers for the first time since July.

Application was made to the MHRT in November and independent psychiatric reports were obtained recommending HL's discharge. Before a MHRT hearing application was also made for a Managers' Hearing. On December 5 HL was allowed home on Section 17 leave and on December 12 the Managers discharged him from the Section 3.

Procedural safeguards for those detained under the Mental Health Act 1983

The European Court noted the following safeguards:
  (a) statutory criteria need to be met and applied by two doctors and an applicant
  (b) Part IV consent to treatment procedures
  (c) Applications and automatic referrals to MH Review Tribunals
  (d) Nearest relative powers (including discharge powers)
  (e) Section 117 after-care
  (f) The Code of Practice and the Mental Health Act Commission
  (g) Section 132 rights to information.

Decision of the European Court

The key to the decision is The European Convention on Human Rights Article 5 (Right to liberty and security of person):

"No one shall be deprived of their liberty except for specific cases and in accordance with procedure prescribed by law e.g. after conviction, lawful arrest on suspicion of having committed an offence, lawful detention of person of unsound mind, to prevent spread of infectious diseases. Everyone deprived of liberty by arrest or detention shall be entitled to take proceedings by which the lawfulness of the detention shall be decided speedily by a Court and release ordered if the detention is not lawful."

The Court concluded that HL was "deprived of his liberty" within the meaning of Article 5.1. It was not crucial that the door was locked or lockable. "The Court considers the key factor in the present case to be that the health care professionals treating and managing the applicant exercised complete and effective control over his care and movements from the moment he presented acute behavioural problems on 22 July 1997 to the date he was compulsorily detained on 29 October 1997." It was clear that "the applicant would only be released from the hospital to the care of Mr and Mrs E as and when those professionals considered it appropriate." HL "was under continuous supervision and control and was not free to leave."

The Court accepted that HL was suffering from a mental disorder of a kind or degree warranting compulsory confinement. However, the Court found that there had been a breach of Article 5.1 in that there was an absence of procedural safeguards to protect against arbitrary deprivation of liberty in the reliance on the common law doctrine of necessity. Article 5.4 was also breached in that the applicant had no right to have the lawfulness of his detention reviewed speedily by a court. Judicial review and habeas corpus proceedings were not adequate. The Court did not find there had been a breach of Article 14.

Implications

Each case will need to be looked at on its own merits but in a situation similar to that of HL it is unlikely to be safe to rely on the common law especially where the criteria for detention under the Mental Health Act appear to be met. Morgan Cole (health and social care law specialists) gives the following advice in its 13th Mental Health Law Bulletin (available in full at www.morgan-cole.com/health):

"Section 6(1) of the Human Rights Act 1998 requires a "public authority", such as a NHS Trust or a local authority, not to act in a way which is incompatible with a Convention right (an independent hospital which performs functions under the 1983 Act is a "public authority" for the purposes of the 1998 Act). This requirement does not apply if legislation requires the authority to act differently. As the Mental Health Act does not prevent public authorities from protecting the Article 5 rights of mentally incapacitated patients by following the ruling of the ECtHR, all patients who come within the category identified by the ECtHR will have to be the subject of a Mental Health Act assessment. These patients must be:

(i.) mentally incapacitated; and

(ii.) detained in the hospital, i.e. be under the continuous supervision and control of staff and not free to leave.

In terms of freedom to leave, all that is required is for staff to have assessed the patient as being too vulnerable to be allowed to leave: there is no need for this decision to be evidenced by a specific event, such as the refusal of permission for carers to remove the patient from the hospital…

NHS Trusts will need to consider the urgent action they should take at this stage and at what point they should proceed to a formal assessment of patients who may be affected by the ruling. At the very least, it would be sensible for Trusts to identify those patients affected by the judgment who should be the subject of Mental Health Act assessments. Trusts will have to consider whether to await any formal Government Guidance, which it is assumed will be forthcoming, before commencing the assessment process."

Government advice was still not available as at 29th November 2004. In the longer term it remains to be seen whether the Mental Capacity Bill will be robust enough to meet the requirements of Article 5 of the European Convention.

History of mental health legislation

In the ancient world, various safeguards were implemented in respect of people suffering from mental illness at the time of committing an offence. In ancient Egypt, Imhotep (Greek Imouthes) combined the roles of priest, statesman, scientist and physician to the second king of the third dynasty, Djoser, who reigned from 2630 to 2611 BC. The temple of Imhotep became a medical school offering various therapies to patients, such as sleep and occupational therapy, narcotherapy and art therapy.

For the ancient Hebrews, the Torah established cities of refuge for people who had accidentally killed someone (Deuteronomy 19). On entering such a city of refuge, a person guilty of manslaughter would be safe from the revenge of relatives of the victim.

Aristotle argued that a person was morally responsible for their crime only if guilt was present, with the perpetrator deliberately choosing to commit the act.

Offenders were tried in the forum in the ancient Roman world, from which comes our term 'forensic'. The Romans took the view that those who were mad were punished enough by their madness and should not be punished additionally (*satis furore punitor*). Under Roman law, the insane were exempt from the usual punishments for causing injury to others: 'An insane person, as well as an infant, are legally incapable of malicious intent and the power to insult, and therefore the action for injuries cannot be brought against them' (the opinions of Julius Paulus, Book V, Title IV: Concerning Injuries; cited in Formigoni 1996).

That allowance was made in sentencing mentally disordered offenders in England after the fall of the Roman Empire is illustrated by the fact that during the reign of King Alfred, a judge who hanged a madman was himself hanged. However, in the UK, until the nineteenth century, 'lunatics' who committed crimes were sent to jails or houses of correction, where they were grossly neglected, objects of derision and sources of entertainment and amusement for the public.

Within the UK, there are three main separate systems of legislation: for England and Wales, for Scotland, and for Northern Ireland. Therefore, there are three different Mental Health Acts. The Republic of Ireland (Eire) also has separate legislation.

One of the earliest references to legal practice in the UK dealing with the mentally ill was in 1285, when a verdict of misadventure was returned by jurors following the killing of one of the brothers at a hospital in Beverley, Yorkshire, on the grounds that the offender acted at 'the instigation of the devil', as a result of which he had become 'frantic and mad'.

An early distinction in common law between the 'idiot', with significant or severe learning difficulties, and the 'lunatic', who was mentally ill, was made. Subsequently, these two groups were dealt with sometimes separately and at other times together in mental health legislation.

The **Royal Prerogative** (*De Praerogativa Regis*) in 1334 entitled the Crown to the rents and profits of the estates of 'idiots', subject to the expense of their maintenance and that of their dependent family. The care of an 'idiot' was often entrusted by the Crown to someone who shared the profits of the estate with the Crown ('begging a man for a fool'). In the case of 'lunatics', however, income greater than the expense of their maintenance was held in a trust for their recovery or, if they died, for the benefit of their soul.

The Bethlem Hospital was founded in 1247 as the Priory of the Order of St Mary of Bethlehem. By 1329, it was described as a hospice or hospital. It first took 'lunatics' in 1377. It remained the only specialized placement for mentally ill people until the seventeenth century.

Overall, in the sixteenth and seventeenth centuries in England, more concern was taken with men who became insane than with their female counterparts. From this time dates the description of Mad Tom, a beggar with tattered clothes and little better than a beast.

The **Poor Law Act of 1601** required each parish to take responsibility for the old and the sick, including 'idiots' and 'lunatics'. Overseers could arrange for the poor to be placed in workhouses, which were known for their appalling conditions. Mentally disordered patients were among those so housed. By 1770, some workhouses were refusing to take 'lunatics'.

The **1713 and 1744 Vagrancy Acts** allowed for the detention of 'Lunaticks or mad persons'.

The **1713 Vagrancy Act**, 'the Act for … the more effectual punishing such as Rogues, Vagabonds, Sturdy beggars and Vagrants and Sending them Whither They Ought to be sent', came into operation in 1714. It allowed two or more Justices of the Peace to order the arrest of any person 'furiously mad and dangerous' and for such people 'to be safely locked up in some secure place' for as long as the 'lunacy or madness shall continue'. Secure places included workhouses, private madhouses, jails and Bridewell, a house of correction. 'Lunatics', unlike other vagrants, were excluded from whipping.

In the 1730s, the Bethlem Hospital made provision for 'incurables' and in 1739 stated that it would give priority to such people who were dangerous rather than harmless.

The **1744 Vagrancy Act** amended the 1713 Act by specifying that 'those who by Lunacy or otherwise are furiously mad or so far disordered in their Senses that may be dangerous to be permitted to go abroad' could be apprehended by a constable, church warden or overseer of the poor at the authorization of two or more Justices of the Peace 'and be safely locked in some secure place … (and if necessary) to be there chained … for and during such time only as the lunacy or madness shall continue'.

In 1760, Laurence, the fourth Earl Ferrers, committed an act of murder for which he was tried by his fellow peers before the House of Lords. The murder having been proven easily to have been committed by him, as part of his defence Earl Ferrers called several witnesses in order to try to demonstrate that he had been of unsound mind at the time of the index offence. This included the first appearance of a physician at a trial as an expert witness to address the issue of the mental state of a defendant at the time of the offence. (Earl Ferrers commented on the fact that he had been reduced to the necessity of attempting to prove himself a 'lunatic', such that he might not be deemed a murderer.) This defence failed and Earl Ferrers was sentenced to death; his petition to be beheaded also failed, and he was duly hanged on 5 May 1760.

Medical certification for insanity was introduced by the **Act for Regulating Private Madhouses in 1774** and provided for a fine of £100 unless the proprietor of the private madhouse received an individual under 'an Order in Writing under the Hand and Seal of some Physician, Surgeon or Apothecary, that such person is properly received into such house or Place as a Lunatick'. This followed two cases of habeas corpus (Clark in 1718, Turlington in 1761) and the parliamentary investigation of London madhouses in 1763.

Ticehurst opened in 1792. It rapidly attracted the aristocracy and became the most expensive private asylum in England. The Retreat in York was founded by William Tuke and the Society of Friends in 1792.

In 1800, James Hadfield, an ex-soldier who had brain damage from a sword wound to the head, believed he had to sacrifice his life to save the world; feeling unable to commit suicide, he tried, unsuccessfully, to kill King George III, whom he shot in an attempt to ensure his own execution. Hadfield was acquitted of attempted murder, owing mainly to his lawyer, Erskine, and sent to the Bethlem Hospital. Erskine had emphasized to the court to good effect Hadfield's exposed head wound with visibly throbbing blood vessels. This was the first example of a mentally abnormal offender being sent by a court to a mental hospital. This decision reflected the then sympathy for the mentally ill, as George III also suffered from mental illness, probably as a result of an inherited biochemical disorder of haemoglobin, porphyria. The court's decision about Hadfield led in the same year to the **Act for the Safe Custody of Insane Persons Charged with Offences 1800**. This was retrospective legislation providing for the special verdict of not guilty by reason of insanity. Insanity was, however, undefined. The return of this verdict led to the accused being detained in 'strict custody' in the county jail during His Majesty's pleasure. During the first five years of its operation, 37 people were so detained, which led to the complaint that 'to confine such persons in a common jail is equally destructive for the recovery of the insane and for the security and comfort of other prisoners'.

By 1807, there were 45 private madhouses in the country. The **Act for the Better Care and Maintenance of Pauper and Criminal Lunatics 1808** allowed for insane offenders to be admitted to asylums at the expense of the responsible parish. The **Lunacy Asylum Enabling Act 1808** authorized counties to raise rates to build asylums, although few responded initially; some psychiatric hospitals today were developed as a result of this Act. They tended to be built in rural areas away from towns, but this may have reflected the fact that rural areas were where most of the population then lived. This Act is sometimes referred to as the **County Asylums Act of 1808**. Conditions in asylums remained poor. For example, in 1814 Godfrey Higgins, a governor and Yorkshire magistrate, discovered at the York Lunatic Asylum 13 women confined to a cell measuring 3.66 m × 2.39 m; in addition, Higgins claimed that 144 deaths had been covered up at the asylum. A subsequent official investigation by Higgins and the Tukes found evidence of murder and rape, widespread use of chains, huge embezzlement and physical neglect. In 1814, James (William) Norris was discovered in the Bethlem Hospital, where he had been an inpatient for 9 to 14 years in a specially constructed iron restraint encasing his body from the neck down and attached to a short chain running from the ceiling to the floor, which allowed him only to lie on his back and move 30 cm away from the bar. While Norris had a history of past violence, he was found to be rational.

The **Care and Maintenance Lunacy Act of 1815** required overseers of the poor to return lists of 'idiots' and 'lunatics' within parishes, together with certificates from medical practitioners.

The **Madhouse Act of 1828** repealed the 1774 Act. It also increased the number of Metropolitan Commissioners to 15 (including five medical practitioners who received token payments; the rest gave their services free of charge) and gave them the power to release individuals detained improperly and to remove a private madhouse proprietor's licence if conditions were unsatisfactory. This Act also introduced the first legal requirement for medical attendance at least once a week, including signing a weekly register. A medical superintendent had to be employed where an asylum contained more than 100 patients.

The **County Asylums Act 1828** required magistrates to send annual returns of admissions, discharges and deaths to the Home Office. The Act also allowed the Secretary of State to send a visitor to any county asylum, although the visitor had no power to intervene in the administration of that asylum.

The **Poor Law Amendment Act 1834** restricted the period of detention of any dangerous 'lunatic' or insane person or 'idiot' in any workhouse to 14 days, which resulted in dangerous 'lunatics' being admitted to the county asylums and the workhouses retaining the non-dangerous pauper 'lunatics', although workhouse placement of the latter, if curable, was considered unsatisfactory by the Poor Law Commissioners.

Northampton General Lunatic Asylum, a charitable hospital (now St Andrew's Hospital, an independent psychiatric hospital), opened in 1838, taking all county paupers and patients on a contractual basis, including poet John Clare in 1841.

The **Insane Prisoners Act 1840** gave the Home Secretary the power to transfer from prison to an asylum any individual awaiting trial or serving a sentence of imprisonment. This required a certificate of insanity signed by two Justices of the Peace and two doctors.

In 1841, the Association of Medical Officers of Asylums and Hospitals for the Insane was formed, the forerunner of the Royal College of Psychiatrists. The association began publishing its *Asylum Journal* in 1853.

In 1843, Daniel McNaughton, while deluded, attempted to shoot the Prime Minister, Sir Robert Peel. McNaughton missed and shot Peel's secretary instead. McNaughton was acquitted on account of his insanity at the time of the offence. The outcry, including from Queen Victoria, at this acquittal led to the law lords issuing guidance known as the McNaughton Rules, from which the defendant may argue that at the time of the index offence he or she was not guilty by reason of insanity. Further details of the McNaughton Rules are given in Chapter 5.

The **Lunatics Act 1845** introduced detailed certification processes with increased safeguards against the wrongful detention of patients in both public and private facilities. All asylums were ordered to keep a Medical Visitation Book and a record of medical treatment for each patient in a Medical Casebook. This allowed a person who signed an order for admission of a private patient to discharge that patient, although this could be barred by the medical person in charge of the house or a registered medical attendant by certifying that such an individual was 'dangerous and unfit to be at large', which in turn could be overruled by the written consent of the Commissioners in Lunacy. It was also this 1845 Act that introduced the concept of person of unsound mind.

The **Lunatics Asylum Act 1845** required all boroughs and counties to provide within three years adequate asylum accommodation for their pauper 'lunatics' at public expense. Counties were also authorized, but not instructed, to erect less costly buildings for chronic 'lunatics'. The subsequent development of county asylums is reflected by the fact that of 52 counties, 15 had made provision for the insane in 1844, 36 by 1847, and 41 by 1854.

The **Lunatics Act 1853** required medical officers to record in the medical journal of patients the means of, duration of and reasons for restraint and seclusion, or otherwise face a £20 fine. The rules of every asylum had to be given formally to the Home Secretary for approval, although approval was, in fact, undertaken by the Lunacy Commission. The rules were to be 'printed, abided by and observed'. The Bethlem Hospital was also brought under the control of the Lunacy Commission by this Act.

In 1854, the hypodermic syringe was invented.

The **Medical Registration Act 1858** united the medical profession, which previously had been separated into physicians, surgeons and apothecaries.

The Select Committee on Lunacy 1859–60 extended the requirement for an order from a magistrate to detain a 'lunatic' to private, and not just pauper, cases to protect 'the liberty of the subject' and to check on the medical opinion. It also recommended emergency certification and the 'terminalability of orders' to reduce the population of asylums.

Although the Bethlem Hospital had been given money to take mentally disordered offenders, the resulting stigma felt by the hospital led to the **Criminal Lunatic Asylum Act 1860**, under which such offenders were to be placed in a new state criminal lunatic asylum, which opened in 1863 and was later renamed Broadmoor Hospital, the first of the special hospitals.

An **Act to Amend the Law relating to Lunatics 1862** resulted in the cost of caring for 'lunatics' being chargeable upon a common fund of the union of parishes instead of upon an individual parish.

The Annual Report of the Lunacy Commission in 1862 indicated that, by this time, mechanical restraint was used in very few places and on very few occasions. Seclusion was, however, noted to be used in most asylums.

In 1882, paraldehyde was developed.

The **Idiots Act 1886** was the first time that legislation had addressed specifically the needs of people with learning disabilities. Previously, such people had been admitted to workhouses, lunatic asylums and prisons. This Act led to the admission of these people to specialized asylums, such as the previously established 'asylum for idiots' at Park House, Highgate, later known as Earlswood Asylum, and to the regulation and inspection of such asylums. This legislation introduced separate provisions for 'idiots' and 'imbeciles'.

The distinction between 'idiots' and 'imbeciles' was, however, ignored by the **Lunacy (Consolidation) Act 1890**, which favoured public over private provision and provided for four routes of admission:

- *Summary reception order*: pauper patients were usually received under this order following a Justice of the Peace being petitioned by a police officer or a Poor Law relieving officer with a medical certificate. In an emergency, a wandering 'lunatic' could be detained in a workhouse for up to three days by one of these officers.
- *Reception order*: non-pauper patients were usually admitted under this order. For this, a magistrates' or county court judge was petitioned to order admission by a relative, preferably the patient's spouse, supported by two medical certificates, one of which, if practical, should be from the individual's usual medical attendant. The relative was legally required to visit the patient at least once every six months.
- *Urgency order*: private patients could be admitted following a petition from a relative to the asylum authorities in an emergency for up to seven days under this order, following which a reception order was to be obtained, otherwise the patient would be discharged.
- *Chancery lunatics*: such patients could be admitted by a process of application for admission following inquisition.

Reception orders lasted for up to one year, but they were renewable if the manager of the institution provided a special report and a certificate to the Lunacy Commission, which, if it accepted the opinion of the report, renewed the order for a further year, thereafter for two and then three years, and then for successive periods of five years. If not satisfied, the Lunacy Commission retained the power directly to discharge such patients from asylums. Indeed, one medical commissioner and one legal commissioner together could discharge a patient from any hospital or licensed house after one visit.

Also under the Lunacy Act 1890, with permission of the Lunacy Commission or the licensing justices, managers of licensed houses could receive as boarders 'any person who is desirous of voluntarily submitting to treatment', but they too had to be produced to the Lunacy Commission and the justices on their visits. Such voluntary patients could leave after giving 24 hours' notice. Detention beyond this rendered the proprietor liable to a daily £10 fine. However, the consent of the commissioners and licensing justices was still required, and boarders were confined largely to licensed houses.

In 1895, Josef Breuer and Sigmund Freud published their *Studies on Hysteria* (*Studien über Hysterie*), detailing their cathartic model of treatment.

In 1896, the National Association for the Care of the Feeble Minded was founded.

In 1900, Freud's *The Interpretation of Dreams* was published, with its topographical model of the unconscious, pre-conscious and conscious levels of the mind.

In 1912, the new Rampton State Asylum opened as a criminal lunatic asylum in the village of Woodbeck, north Nottinghamshire. Initially, all patients were transferred from Broadmoor Hospital. Later, the asylum also took people with learning disabilities and requiring a special hospital placement. It remains one of the three maximum secure special hospitals in England.

The **Mental Deficiency Act 1913** followed the by then current opinion favouring the segregation of 'mental defectives' into four legal classes:

- *idiots*, who were unable to guard themselves against common physical dangers such as fire, water or traffic;

- *imbeciles*, who could guard against physical dangers but were incapable of managing themselves or their affairs;
- the *feeble-minded*, who needed care or control for the protection of self or others;
- *moral defectives*, who had vicious or criminal propensities. This category was, in fact, also used to include and detain many poor women with illegitimate or unsupported babies.

This Act also founded a Board of Control and placed on local government the responsibility for the supervision and protection of such individuals, both in institutions and in the community. Also under this Act, local authorities were given statutory responsibility for providing occupation and training for 'mental defectives'.

The **Ministry of Health Act 1919** transferred responsibility for the Board of Control from the Home Office to the newly formed Ministry of Health.

In 1923, Freud's *The Ego and the Id* was published, with its structural model of the mind involving id, ego and superego, together with eros, the life instinct, and thanatos, the death instinct.

In 1926, the Report of the Royal Commission on Lunacy and Mental Disorder (Macmillan) recommended that madness be defined in medical terms. It commented that compulsion was becoming less appropriate. In the same year, the annual report of the Board of Control saw the first official use of the term 'community care'.

The **Mental Deficiency Act 1927** gave more emphasis to care outside the institutions. Mental deficiency was defined as 'a condition of arrested or incomplete development of mind existing before the age of 18 years whether arising from inherent causes or induced by disease or injury'.

The **Mental Treatment Act 1930** allowed for informal voluntary admission and represented the turning point from legal to medical control of psychiatric admissions. 'Lunatics' became 'persons of unsound mind' and asylums became 'mental hospitals'. Voluntary admission was by written application to the person in charge of the hospital, but magistrates continued to be involved in overseeing compulsory hospital admissions. The Act also allowed local authorities to establish psychiatric outpatient clinics in both general and mental hospitals and organize aftercare for discharged patients, but services remained centred on the mental hospital.

Insulin coma therapy was invented by the Austrian psychiatrist Manfred Joshua Sakel in 1935. Psycho-surgery (leucotomy) as a treatment of mental illness was established by Egas Moniz in Portugal in 1935, being used in the UK for the first time in Bristol in 1940. In 1934, convulsive therapy by drugs, e.g. camphor, was introduced in Hungary by Ladislas von Meduna, reaching the UK in 1937. Electrically induced convulsion (electroconvulsive therapy, ECT) was first undertaken in 1938 by two Italians, Hugo Cerletti and Lucio Beni, on a mute man who suffered from schizophrenia (in contrast to its main use now in severe depression). The patient's first words after his initial treatment were 'You are killing me', but the treatments were continued and the man's mental state improved. ECT was first used in the UK the following year. Also in the late 1930s, amphetamines were used to treat depression. Psychiatric wards started to become unlocked in the UK in the 1930s and 1940s.

The **National Health Service Act 1946** ended the distinction between paying and non-paying patients.

Also in 1946, Judy Fryd, a mother of a child with a learning disability, formed the National Association of Parents of Backward Children. This association changed its name to the National Society for Mentally Handicapped Children in 1956, and then to Mencap in the 1960s.

The **National Assistance Act 1948** made provisions for those in need.

D-Lysergic acid diethylamide (LSD) was used in a therapeutic trial in 1952 when Sandoz supplied Powick Hospital in Worcestershire with the drug. (LSD-25 had been synthesized in 1938 by Albert Hofmann, a chemist working for Sandoz. The first (accidental) human experience of the effects of this chemical was by Hofmann in 1943, when he reported seeing 'an uninterrupted stream of fantastic pictures'.

Chlorpromazine (sold as Largactil in the UK and as Thorazine in the USA) was first marketed as an antipsychotic medication in Great Britain in 1954. In 1956, clinical studies confirmed the effectiveness in treating depression of both the monoamine oxidase inhibitor iproniazid, which was first used in 1952 in tuberculosis causing euphoria in some of those so treated, and the tricyclic antidepressant imipramine.

The Percy Commission, the Royal Commission on the Law relating to Mental Illness and Mental Deficiency, was appointed in 1953. Its report in 1957 formed the basis for the new **Mental Health Act 1959 in England and Wales** as well as the **Mental Health (Scotland) Act 1960** and the **Mental Health (Northern Ireland) Act in 1961**.

The **Mental Health Act 1959** led to voluntary informal admissions being the usual method of psychiatric hospital admission. No longer was a positive statement of such willingness to be admitted on the part of the patient required. All judicial controls on compulsory admission were removed. Applications for admissions were to be made by a mental welfare officer (social worker) or by the patient's nearest relative. Mental disorder was defined as including mental illness, severe subnormality, subnormality and psychopathic disorder. Provisions included a 28-day compulsory order for admission for observation (Section 25), which was non-renewable and required two medical certificates; a 72-hour emergency order (Section 29) on the basis of one medical certificate, which could be converted by the addition of a further medical certificate into an order for observation; and a treatment order (Section 26) for a maximum period of 12 months in the first instance, on the basis of two medical certificates, renewable after 12 months and thereafter for periods of two years. Appeals to a Mental Health Review Tribunal were allowed once in the first period of detention and once in each period for which detention was renewed.

In 1961, Minister of Health J. Enoch Powell announced that 'in 15 years' time there would be needed not more than half as many places in hospital for mental illness as there are today', which would represent '75 000' fewer hospital beds.

Haloperidol, an oral antipsychotic medication, was introduced in 1959.

The 1962 White Paper, Hospital Plan for England and Wales, proposed the creation of new and large district general hospitals but made no specific reference to provision for long-stay psychiatric patients. The Seebohm Report of 1968 noted that community care was, for many parts of the country, a 'sad illusion' and was likely to remain so for many years ahead.

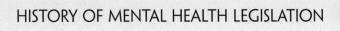
The Royal College of Psychiatrists received its charter in 1971.

In 1975, the Butler Committee Report on Mentally Abnormal Offenders recommended the establishment of regional (medium) secure units, pending the development of which temporary interim secure units were to be established in each region.

The **Local Authorities Social Services Act 1970** created social services departments. In the same year, the **Chronically Sick and Disabled Persons Act 1970** was passed, which also applied to mentally disordered people.

In 1980, the Boynton Report of the Review of Rampton Hospital was published. This followed allegations of abuse at this special hospital that had been made in a Yorkshire Television documentary, *The Secret Hospital.*

The Mental Health (Amendment) Act of 1982, introduced as a Bill in November 1981, led to the **Mental Health Act 1983 for England and Wales**. Under this Act, voluntary admissions were still to be encouraged, but the legislation was more legalistic in its approach to mental health. Changes were made to the definition of mental disorder. Mental disorder was defined as including mental illness (which was undefined), severe mental impairment and mental impairment (which replaced subnormality), and psychopathic disorder. (The corresponding 1984 Scottish Mental Health Act uses the term 'mental handicap' rather than 'mental impairment'.) The Mental Health Act 1983 also introduced a separate treatability test for psychopathic disorder and mental impairment. Detention orders were effectively halved in length and opportunities to apply for a Mental Health Review Tribunal hearing doubled. Tribunal hearings were to be made available to 28-day assessment order (Section 2) patients. Also introduced were powers for a Mental Health Review Tribunal to order delayed discharge and to recommend, but not order, leave of absence or transfer. Tribunals, when chaired by a judge or Queen's Counsel (QC or 'Silk'), could now also discharge from restriction orders (Section 42), which previously only the Home Secretary could do. Provisions for consent to treatment were specified, and the Mental Health Act Commission was introduced. There were also changes to guardianship and a requirement for training of social workers before appointment as approved social workers under the Act. Informal inpatients were allowed to retain voting rights and access to the courts and were also entitled to the provision of aftercare services (Section 117). The proposed Mental Health Act Code of Practice was eventually laid before Parliament in December 1989 (pursuant to Section 118(4) of the Mental Health Act 1983) and published in 1990.

The **Police and Criminal Evidence Act 1984** (PACE) with its code of practice used the term 'mental disorder' as in the 1983 Mental Health Act, and the term 'mental handicap', defined as 'a state of arrested or incomplete development of mind which includes significant impairment of intelligence and social functioning'.

In the late 1980s, newer classes of safer antidepressants were marketed, including the selective serotonin reuptake inhibitors (SSRIs), such as fluvoxamine (marketed as Faverin) and fluoxetine (marketed as Prozac).

In 1989, Ashworth Special Hospital was formed when two Liverpool special hospitals in close proximity were amalgamated – Moss Side Hospital, which had opened in 1919, and Park Lane Hospital, which had opened in 1974. In the same year, a new authority, the Special Hospitals Service Authority, took charge of Broadmoor, Ashworth and Rampton special hospitals.

Clozapine, an oral atypical antipsychotic medication for treatment-resistant schizophrenia, was re-introduced in 1990, with strict requirements for blood monitoring after its original failed introduction owing to mortality from induced low white cell counts in the 1970s.

In 1990, the **National Health Service and Community Care Act 1990** was introduced.

The Care-Programme Approach Circular was published in 1990, which was to take effect from April 1991. The issue of the adequacy of community care was highlighted by the killing by Christopher Clunes, who suffered from schizophrenia, of Jonathon Zito at Finsbury Park tube station in London in December 1992 and also, on New Year's Day 1993, by Ben Silcock, then aged 27 years and who also suffered from schizophrenia, who climbed into the lions' enclosure at London Zoo and was severely mauled and injured by the animals.

A revised Mental Health Code of Practice came into effect in November 1993 following publication in August of that year. The Secretary of State for Health, Virginia Bottomley, introduced a ten-point plan for the care of mentally disordered people.

In April 1995, the publication of HSG (94)(5) heralded the introduction of supervision registers in October 1994, which have now become largely obsolete. The Department of Health published *Building Bridges: A Guide to Inter-agency Working* in November 1995.

The **Mental Health (Patients in the Community) Act 1995**, with its provisions for supervised discharge/aftercare under supervision, came into effect in April 1996.

In September 1998, Professor Genevra Richardson of Queen Mary and Westfield College, London, was appointed to lead a root-and-branch review of the Mental Health Act 1983. The expert committee, chaired by Professor Richardson, reported to ministers at the Department of Health in July 1999, having consulted a wide range of organizations and individuals in formulating their proposals. They issued their Draft Outline Proposals to over 350 key stakeholders to consider the practicability of the proposals. In 1999, the Report of the Expert Committee was published.

In 2002, a Draft Mental Health Bill was published by the Department of Health. In 2004, a Revised Draft Mental Health Bill was published.

FURTHER READING

Fennell, P (1996). *Treatment Without Consent: Law, Psychiatry and Treatment of Mentally Disordered People since 1845.* London: Routledge.

Formigoni, W (1996). *Pithanon a Paulo Epitomatorum libri VIII: Sulla funzione critica del commento del giurista Iulius Paulus.* Milan: Giuffrè.

Scull, A (1993). *The Most Solitary of Afflictions: Madness in Society in Britain 1700–1900.* London: Yale University Press.

Definitions used in mental health legislation

The definition of mental disorder for the purposes of the Act is set out in Section 1 of the Mental Health Act. Other definitions are given in Section 145. Definitions used in Part III of the Act (patients concerned in criminal proceedings or under sentence) are not considered in this chapter but can be found in Chapter 5.

MENTAL DISORDER

The Mental Health Act sets out in Section 1 a broader definition of the term 'mental disorder' and then four specific categories within.

Broad definition

The term 'mental disorder' means:

- mental illness (see below);
- arrested or incomplete development of mind;
- psychopathic disorder (see below);
- any other disorder or disability of mind.

The term 'mentally disordered' is construed according to the above definition.

Relevant sections for broad definition

The broad definition given above is the relevant definition for the following sections of the Mental Health Act:

- Section 2: admission for assessment;
- Section 4: admission for assessment in cases of emergency;
- Section 5(2): doctor's holding power;
- Section 5(4): nurse's holding power;
- Section 131: informal admission;

- Section 135: warrant to search for and remove patients;
- Section 136: police powers to remove persons from public places.

Arrested or incomplete development of mind

The term 'arrested or incomplete development of mind' corresponds to the term 'mental handicap' used in the **Police and Criminal Evidence Act 1984** and covers a number of people with significant learning disabilities. Guidance given on the use of this term in the Code of Practice (Department of Health and Welsh Office 1999, Paragraph 30.5) is as follows:

> This implies that the features that determine the learning disability were present at some stage which permanently prevented the usual maturation of intellectual and social development. It excludes persons whose learning disability derives from accident, injury or illness occurring after that point usually accepted as complete development.

There is no age specified, but if the cause of the mental disability were an accident as an adult after 'complete development', then this would be excluded from this definition. This would also exclude such a person from the definitions of mental impairment and severe mental impairment (see below). This would be a problem where such a person needed long-term detention or guardianship (see Chapter 4); he or she could be included under *any other disorder or disability of mind.*

Specific definition

The following four specific categories of mental disorder are given:

- mental illness;
- severe mental impairment;
- mental impairment;
- psychopathic disorder.

Relevant sections for specific definition

A patient must be considered to be suffering from one of the above four specific forms of mental disorder before he or she can be dealt with under the following sections:

- Section 3: admission for treatment;
- Section 7: reception into guardianship;
- Section 25: supervised discharge;
- Section 35: remand to hospital for report on accused's mental condition;
- Section 36: remand to hospital for treatment (only for mental illness or severe mental impairment);
- Section 37: court order for hospital admission or guardianship;
- Section 38: interim hospital order;
- Section 47: transfer to hospital of people serving sentences of imprisonment, etc.

- Section 48: removal to hospital of other prisoners (only for mental illness or severe mental impairment).

Severe mental impairment

This means a state of arrested or incomplete development of mind, which includes severe impairment of intelligence and social functioning. It is associated with abnormally aggressive or seriously irresponsible conduct. The term 'severely mentally impaired' is construed according to this definition.

Mental impairment

This means a state of arrested or incomplete development of mind (not amounting to severe mental impairment), which includes significant impairment of intelligence and social functioning. It is associated with abnormally aggressive or seriously irresponsible conduct. The term 'mentally impaired' is construed according to this definition.

Psychopathic disorder

This means a persistent disorder or disability of mind (whether or not including significant impairment of intelligence) that results in abnormally aggressive or seriously irresponsible conduct.

Exclusions

So far as the definition of mental disorder is concerned, the Act states that a person may not be dealt with under the Mental Health Act as suffering from mental disorder by reason only of:

- promiscuity
- other immoral conduct
- sexual deviancy
- dependence on alcohol
- dependence on drugs.

Mental illness

It should be noted that the Mental Health Act does not define the term 'mental illness'; its operational definition is a matter of clinical judgement in each individual case.

OTHER DEFINITIONS

Absent without leave

This refers to a patient being absent without permission from any hospital or other place and being liable to be taken into custody and returned under Section 18 of the Mental Health Act. Specifically, Section 18 states that a patient who at the time is liable to be detained under Part II of the Mental Health Act in a hospital is considered to be absent without leave if any of the following applies:

- the patient absents him- or herself without leave granted under Section 17 of the Mental Health Act (often referred to as 'Section 17 leave'; see Chapter 4);
- the patient fails to return to the hospital upon being recalled under Section 17;
- the patient fails to return to the hospital at the end of 'Section 17 leave';
- the patient absents him- or herself without permission from any place at which he or she is required to reside under Section 17.

Approved social worker

An approved social worker is an officer of a local social services authority appointed to act as an approved social worker for the purposes of the Mental Health Act. Note that a social worker employed by a private hospital is not an officer of a local social services authority and, therefore, cannot be an approved social worker.

Hospital

This means:

- any health-service hospital within the meaning of the National Health Service Act 1977;
- any accommodation provided by a local authority and used as a hospital by or on behalf of the Secretary of State under the National Health Service Act 1977.

Managers

Hospital

In relation to a hospital as defined above, the term 'the managers' usually refers to the board of the National Health Service (NHS) Trust responsible for the administration of the hospital. The board may set up a special committee to undertake the Trust's duties and responsibilities under the Act.

High-security hospital (special hospital)

In relation to a high-security hospital (see below), the term 'the managers' refers to the Secretary of State.

Registered mental nursing home

In relation to a mental nursing home registered under the Registered Homes Act 1984, the term 'the managers' refers to the person or people registered in respect of the home.

Medical treatment

Under the Mental Health Act, medical treatment includes:

■ nursing;
■ care under medical supervision;
■ habilitation under medical supervision;
■ rehabilitation under medical supervision.

Nearest relative

A relative means the person identified in Section 26 who has certain rights, and includes the following:

■ husband or wife
■ son or daughter
■ parent
■ brother or sister
■ grandparent
■ grandchild
■ uncle or aunt
■ nephew or niece.

For the purposes of the definition of nearest relative:

■ half-blood relationships are treated in the same way as whole-blood relationships;
■ an illegitimate person is treated as the legitimate child of his or her mother and (if the person's father has parental responsibility for him or her under Section 3 of the Children Act 1989) his or her father.

With the exceptions given below, the nearest relative is defined as being the surviving person first described in the above list, with preference being given to:

■ whole-blood relations over half-blood relations;
■ the elder or eldest of two or more relatives at a given position in the list, regardless of sex.

Preference is also given to a relative with whom the patient ordinarily resides or by whom he or she is cared for.

Exceptions

Where the person who would be the nearest relative under the above definition

■ in the case of a patient ordinarily resident in the UK, the Channel Islands or the Isle of Man, is not so resident; or
■ is the husband or wife of the patient but is separated permanently from the patient, either by agreement or under a court order, or has deserted or been deserted by the patient for a period that has not come to an end; or

- is a person other than the husband, wife, father or mother of the patient and is under 18 years of age,

then the nearest relative is determined as if that person were dead.

Spouse

The terms 'husband' and 'wife' include the common-law husband and common-law wife so long as he or she has been living with the patient for at least six months. However, this does not apply to a person living as the patient's spouse if the patient is married, unless the legal spouse is separated permanently from the patient, either by agreement or under a court order, or has deserted or been deserted by the patient for a period that has not come to an end.

Other non-relatives

A person other than a relative with whom the patient has been residing ordinarily for at least five years is treated as a relative who comes last in the above list of relatives. In the case of a married patient, this non-relative cannot count as the nearest relative unless the patient's spouse can be disregarded by virtue of permanent separation or desertion (as outlined above).

Patient

A patient is a person suffering from, or appearing to be suffering from, mental disorder.

Responsible medical officer

Detention under Section 2 or Section 3

In relation to a patient detained under Section 2 or Section 3 of the Mental Health Act, the responsible medical officer is the registered medical practitioner in charge of the treatment of the patient. He or she is usually a consultant psychiatrist.

Guardianship

In relation to a patient subject to guardianship, the responsible medical officer is the medical officer authorized by the local social services authority to act (either generally or in any particular case or for any particular purpose) as the responsible medical officer.

High-security hospital

The traditional term for high-security hospital in England is 'special hospital'. Under Section 4 of the National Health Service Act 1977, a special hospital is defined as being an establishment for:

… persons subject to detention under the Mental Health Act 1983 who in the Secretary of State's opinion require treatment under conditions of special security on account of their dangerous, violent or criminal propensities.

At the time of writing, there are three high-security hospitals in England: Broadmoor, Ashworth and Rampton.

REFERENCE

Department of Health and Welsh Office (1999). *Mental Health Act 1983: Code of Practice.* London: The Stationery Office.

3

Compulsory admission to hospital

Compulsory admission to hospital is covered in Part II of the Mental Health Act under sections 2, 3 and 4.

SECTION 2

Purpose

The purpose of Section 2 is an admission to hospital for assessment.

Grounds and procedure for admission

The grounds for admission under Section 2 are that:

- the patient is suffering from mental disorder of a nature or degree that warrants his or her detention in a hospital for assessment (or for assessment followed by medical treatment) for at least a limited period; *and*
- the patient ought to be so detained in the interests of his or her own health or safety; *or*
- the patient ought to be so detained with a view to the protection of other people.

The procedure for admission under Section 2 is as follows.

- The application preferably should be made by an approved social worker (although the patient's nearest relative can make the application).
- If the applicant is an approved social worker, then he or she must inform the patient's nearest relative that the application is being (or has been) made, either before or within a reasonable time of making the application. The nearest relative cannot prevent this application from being made.
- The applicant (approved social worker or nearest relative) must have seen the patient within the past 14 days.

- Two registered medical practitioners (at least one of whom is approved under Section 12 of the Mental Health Act) must examine the patient within five days of each other and give their signed written recommendations on the appropriate form (see Appendix V).

Duration

Up to 28 days, beginning with the day of admission. The patient must not be detained after the expiration of this period unless before it has expired he or she has become liable to be detained under some other provision of the Mental Health Act.

Discharge

The patient may be discharged by any of the following:

- the responsible medical officer (RMO)
- the hospital managers
- the nearest relative.

Discharge by the nearest relative may, under Section 25 of the Act, be blocked by the hospital managers if the doctor in charge of the case certifies that the patient needs to remain in hospital. In this case, the nearest relative may make an application to a Mental Health Review Tribunal within 28 days. Section 25 of the Act is as follows:

1 An order for discharge of a patient who is liable to be detained in a hospital shall not be made by his nearest relative except after giving not less than 72 hours' notice in writing to the managers of the hospital; and if, within 72 hours after such notice has been given, the responsible medical officer furnishes to the managers a report certifying that in the opinion of that officer the patient, if discharged, would be likely to act in a manner dangerous to other persons or to himself
   (a) any order for the discharge of the patient made by that relative in pursuance of the notice shall be of no effect; and
   (b) no further order for the discharge of the patient shall be made by that relative during the period of six months beginning with the date of the report.
2 In any case where a report under subsection (1) above is furnished in respect of a patient who is liable to be detained in pursuance of an application for admission for treatment the managers shall cause the nearest relative of the patient to be informed.

The patient may make an application to a Mental Health Review Tribunal within 14 days of being detained under Section 2.

Pointers to compulsory admission under Section 2 rather than Section 3

It can sometimes be difficult to decide whether to use Section 2 or Section 3 (see below). Chapter 5 of the Code of Practice advises applying professional judgement to the criteria in each section and gives the following pointers to using Section 2 rather than Section 3:

- where the diagnosis and prognosis of a patient's condition are unclear;
- where there is a need to carry out an inpatient assessment in order to formulate a treatment plan;
- where a judgement is needed as to whether the patient will accept treatment on a voluntary basis following admission;
- where a judgement has to be made as to whether a particular treatment proposal, which can be administered to the patient only under Part IV of the Act, is likely to be effective;
- where a patient who has already been assessed, and who previously has been admitted compulsorily under the Act, is judged to have changed since the previous admission and needs further assessment;
- where the patient previously has not been admitted to hospital, either compulsorily or informally.

Note that the nearest relative can block an application for compulsory admission under Section 3 but cannot do so for an application for compulsory admission under Section 2. According to Paragraph 5.4 of the Code of Practice, decisions as to whether to choose Section 2 or Section 3 should not be influenced by any of the following:

- wanting to avoid consulting the nearest relative;
- the fact that a proposed treatment to be administered under the Act will last less than 28 days;
- the fact that a patient detained under Section 2 will get quicker access to a Mental Health Review Tribunal than will a patient detained under Section 3.

SECTION 3

Purpose

Section 3 is an admission to hospital for treatment.

Grounds and procedure for admission

An application for admission for treatment may be made in respect of a patient on the grounds that:

(a) he is suffering from mental illness, severe mental impairment, psychopathic disorder or mental impairment *and* his mental disorder is of a nature or degree which makes it appropriate for him to receive medical treatment in a hospital; *and*

(b) in the case of psychopathic disorder or mental impairment, such treatment is likely to alleviate or prevent a deterioration of his condition; *and*

(c) it is necessary for the health or safety of the patient *or* for the protection of other persons that he should receive such treatment *and* it cannot be provided unless he is detained under this section.

The application preferably should be made by an approved social worker (although the nearest relative can make the application).

If the applicant is an approved social worker, he or she must consult the nearest relative if at all possible. Under Section 11(4):

> ... no such application shall be made by such a social worker except after consultation with the person (if any) appearing to be the nearest relative of the patient unless it appears to that social worker that in the circumstances such consultation is not reasonably practicable or would involve unreasonable delay.

The nearest relative can prevent this application being made. Under Section 11(4):

> Neither an application for admission for treatment nor a guardianship application shall be made by an approved social worker if the nearest relative of the patient has notified that social worker, or the local social services authority by whom that social worker is appointed, that he objects to the application being made ...

If the nearest relative does exercise his or her right to prevent this application being made, then, if the admission is deemed necessary, the applicant may apply to a court. Under Section 29 of the Act, an acting nearest relative may be appointed by the county court. An application for such an order under Section 29 may be made upon any of the following grounds:

(a) that the patient has no nearest relative within the meaning of this Act, or that it is not reasonably practicable to ascertain whether he has such a relative, or who that relative is;

(b) that the nearest relative of the patient is incapable of acting as such by reason of mental disorder or other illness;

(c) that the nearest relative of the patient unreasonably objects to the making of an application for admission for treatment or a guardianship application in respect of the patient; or

(d) that the nearest relative of the patient has exercised without due regard to the welfare of the patient or the interests of the public his power to discharge the patient from hospital or guardianship under Part II of the Act, or is likely to do so.

The applicant (approved social worker or nearest relative) must have seen the patient within the past 14 days.

Two registered medical practitioners (at least one of whom is approved under the Mental Health Act) must examine the patient within five days of each other and give their signed written recommendations on the appropriate form (see Appendix V).

Duration

Up to six months. The RMO may renew the Section 3 for a further six months and then annually.

Discharge

The patient may be discharged by any of the following:

- the RMO
- the hospital managers
- the nearest relative (who must give 72 hours' notice).

Discharge by the nearest relative may be blocked under Section 25 of the Act if, within 72 hours after the nearest relative has given notice in writing to the hospital managers that he or she wishes the patient to be discharged, the RMO furnishes to the managers a report certifying that in the opinion of that officer, the patient, if discharged, would be likely to act in a manner dangerous to other people or to him- or herself. In this case, the nearest relative may make an application to a Mental Health Review Tribunal for the patient's discharge within 28 days of being informed of this decision.

The patient may make an application to a Mental Health Review Tribunal within six months of being detained under Section 3. If the patient does not do so and is further detained under this section, then the hospital managers must automatically refer the patient to a Mental Health Review Tribunal.

Pointers to compulsory admission under Section 3 rather than Section 2

It can sometimes be difficult to decide whether to use Section 3 or Section 2 (see above). Chapter 5 of the Code of Practice advises applying professional judgement to the criteria in each section and gives the following pointers to using Section 3 rather than Section 2:

(a) where a patient has been admitted in the past, is considered to need compulsory admission for the treatment of a mental disorder which is already known to his clinical team, and has been assessed in the recent past by that team;

(b) where a patient already admitted under Section 2 who is assessed as needing further medical treatment for mental disorder under the Act at the conclusion of his detention under Section 2 is unwilling to remain in hospital informally and to consent to the medical treatment;

(c) where a patient is detained under Section 2 and assessment points to a need for treatment under the Act for a period beyond the 28-day detention under Section 2. In such circumstances an application for detention under Section 3 should be made at the earliest opportunity and should not be delayed until the end of Section 2 detention. Such action may well deprive the patient of an opportunity to apply to a Mental Health Review Tribunal under Section 2. (Where such action is taken, then managers should consider reviewing the patient's detention quickly.)

Note that the nearest relative can block an application for compulsory admission under Section 3 but cannot do so for an application for compulsory admission under Section 2. According to Paragraph 5.4 of the Code of Practice, decisions as to whether to choose Section 2 or Section 3 should not be influenced by any of the following:

- wanting to avoid consulting the nearest relative;
- the fact that a proposed treatment to be administered under the Act will last less than 28 days;
- the fact that a patient detained under Section 2 will get quicker access to a Mental Health Review Tribunal than will a patient detained under Section 3.

SECTION 4

Purpose

The purpose of Section 4 is an admission to hospital for assessment in cases of emergency. This section should be used only in cases of urgent necessity. An application made under this section is referred to as an 'emergency application'.

Grounds and procedure for admission

The grounds for admission under Section 4 are:

- the patient is suffering from mental disorder of a nature or degree that warrants his or her detention in a hospital for assessment (or for assessment followed by medical treatment) for at least a limited period; *and*
- the patient ought to be so detained in the interests of his or her own health or safety; *or* the patient ought to be so detained with a view to the protection of other persons; *and*
- it is of urgent necessity for the patient to be admitted and detained under Section 2; *and*
- compliance with the provisions of the Mental Health Act relating to applications under Section 2 would involve undesirable delay.

The procedure for admission under Section 4 is as follows:

- The application preferably should be made by an approved social worker (although the nearest relative can make the application).
- The applicant (approved social worker or nearest relative) must have seen the patient within the past 24 hours.

- One registered medical practitioner, who, if practicable (but not necessarily if this is not practicable), has had previous acquaintance with the patient (and who need not necessarily be approved under Section 12 of the Mental Health Act if this is not practicable), must examine the patient. The doctor must give his or her signed written recommendation on the appropriate form (see Appendix V).
- The patient must be admitted to hospital within 24 hours of either the medical examination or the application, whichever is earlier.

Duration

Seventy-two hours from the time of admission.

Discharge

By the end of 72 hours, one of the following must be implemented:

- the patient is discharged;
- the patient remains admitted informally;
- a second medical recommendation is received, which, together with the first medical recommendation, allows the requirements for detention under Section 2 to be complied with;
- application for compulsory admission under Section 3 is initiated;
- there is no right to apply to a Mental Health Review Tribunal.

GOOD PRACTICE

The Mental Health Commissioners recommend that, whenever possible, two doctors should be involved in the decision to admit a patient to hospital under the Mental Health Act. That is, sections 2 and 3 should always be used in preference to Section 4 (for which only one doctor is required). They recommend further that the use of Section 4 should be confined to emergencies when it is possible to secure the attendance of only one doctor (Puri and Bermingham 1990).

According to the Code of Practice (Paragraph 6.1), an applicant cannot seek admission for assessment under Section 4 unless:

- the criteria for admission for assessment are met; *and*
- the matter is of urgent necessity; *and*
- there is not enough time to obtain a second medical recommendation.

Section 4 is for genuine emergencies and should never be used for administrative convenience (Department of Health and Welsh Office 1990, Chapter 6).

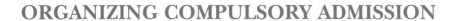

ORGANIZING COMPULSORY ADMISSION

Procedure for general practitioners

Once it is clear that a patient requires admission for psychiatric assessment and/or treatment, the general practitioner (GP) should first attempt to persuade the patient to be admitted informally. If the patient does not protest against this, then the informal admission may be organized in the usual way by contacting the duty psychiatrist.

If the patient refuses informal admission, then he or she will need to be assessed for compulsory admission. The GP should contact the approved social worker; it is the latter who applies for compulsory admission under the Mental Health Act. The local hospital switchboard, police station or social services department will have details of the on-call approved social worker. Although, under the Mental Health Act, the nearest relative can be the applicant, the Code of Practice makes it clear that the approved social worker is usually the right applicant. In most circumstances, the GP should therefore advise the nearest relative that it is preferable for the approved social worker to make an assessment of the need for the patient to be admitted under the Mental Health Act. If necessary, for example because the approved social worker cannot be contacted, the nearest relative can be advised of his or her right to make an application. However, the nearest relative should never be advised to make the application simply in order to avoid involving an approved social worker in the assessment.

For a patient in the community, the approved social worker will normally contact an approved doctor, carry the relevant forms and generally coordinate the assessment. In the case of a patient already in hospital, the senior house officer (SHO) of the clinical team in charge of the case will usually fulfil this role.

It is important, before the assessment, for the GP to gather as much relevant information as possible about the patient. Clearly this entails perusing the patient's medical notes. In addition, in the case of a patient in the community, this may involve consulting colleagues in the same practice and discussing the case with the patient's relatives and the local psychiatric unit.

Mental health assessment

Particular attention should be paid to evidence relating to the health and/or safety of the patient, the risk of harm to others and unusual behaviour that may be indicative of the presence of mental disorder. The mental health assessment should be arranged in such a way that the participants are able to meet, for example outside the patient's home, for a preliminary discussion regarding the conduct of the assessment. In the case of a patient already in hospital, it is important for the doctor(s) to discuss the case with members of the medical and nursing staff and to peruse all relevant case notes.

According to the Code of Practice, a proper medical examination requires:

- direct personal examination of the patient's mental state, taking into account social, cultural and (where relevant) ethnic contexts;
- consideration of all available relevant medical information, including that in the possession of others, professional or non-professional.

If the patient and doctor cannot understand each other's language, then the doctor should, whenever practicable, have recourse to a professional interpreter, including a professional signer in the case of a patient with hearing difficulties and who understands a sign language. The interpreter or signer should understand the terminology and conduct of psychiatric interviews.

Once the patient has been examined and the relevant forms have been filled in, the application should be addressed to the hospital managers. The doctors additionally may fill in separate forms in order to claim their assessment fees.

'Difficult' patients

Although a variety of problems may arise, most can be pre-empted by taking a few precautions. For instance, it is worth checking whether a bed is booked at the admission unit. Similarly, if the patient is known to be aggressive, then the police may be approached for assistance.

A patient with a previous history of psychiatric admission or with partial insight and who wishes to avoid compulsory admission may attempt to do so in a number of ways. The patient may take flight; if this is assessed as being likely to occur, perhaps because of such an incident in the past, then the doctor can try to prevent it happening by explaining carefully to the patient the benefits of admission. Often, such a patient may recognize, albeit at an unconscious level, the need for admission. Again, as with certain prisoners in forensic psychiatric assessments, a patient in the community may attempt to give a misleading picture of his or her mental state; however, whereas the former may try to feign mental illness, the latter may endeavour to suppress evidence of mental illness, for example by being very guarded in replies to questions or even being electively mute. Such a manoeuvre is very likely to fail, however, if the assessment is thorough and includes interviews with relatives and informants, a consideration of the past history and discussion with others involved in the care of the patient, either previously or at the time of the assessment. It should be noted that muteness may, in itself, be a function of a mental illness, for example severe depression or catatonic schizophrenia. In such cases, other features of the underlying mental illness will be present and can be elicited.

If a person living alone refuses access to his or her home and there is reasonable reason to believe that he or she has been, or is being, ill-treated or neglected, or that he or she is unable to care for him- or herself, for example as the result of auditory hallucinations or persecutory delusions, then an application may be made by an approved social worker to a Justice of the Peace for a warrant to be issued to allow the police to enter, by force if need be, and to search for and remove a patient, under Section 135 of the Mental Health Act. Local authorities issue guidance to approved social workers on how to invoke such a power of entry.

Disagreement between the assessors

There may infrequently be disagreement between the assessors as to whether compulsory admission is indicated. In such cases, it is important that each assessor sets out clearly his or her reasoning during a joint discussion. If there is still no resolution, then the doctor(s) and approved social worker may offer to reassess the patient at a later date. However, it is vital in the event of a decision against compulsory admission that an alternative package of care is implemented to ensure continued support for both the patient and his or her family. The patient should also be encouraged to attend a psychiatric outpatient appointment made for the earliest date possible.

REFERENCES

Department of Health and Welsh Office (1999). *Mental Health Act 1983: Code of Practice.* London: The Stationery Office.

Puri, BK, Bermingham, DF (1990). High rate of Section 4 admissions: clinical implications and possible explanation. *Psychiatric Bulletin* **14**, 21–2.

4

Guardianship and supervised aftercare

GUARDIANSHIP

Guardianship, compared with detention, is a little-used part of the Act. However, it is both important and contentious, especially as community-based powers will have a key place in any new legislation. Its use varies considerably in different parts of England and Wales. Generally, use has stabilized after years of increase. From a low base of 60 new guardianships in England in 1983–84, there were 139 new cases in 1988–89 and 669 in 1999–2000. The number of new cases then dipped, and there were 454 new cases in 2002–03. In terms of continuing cases

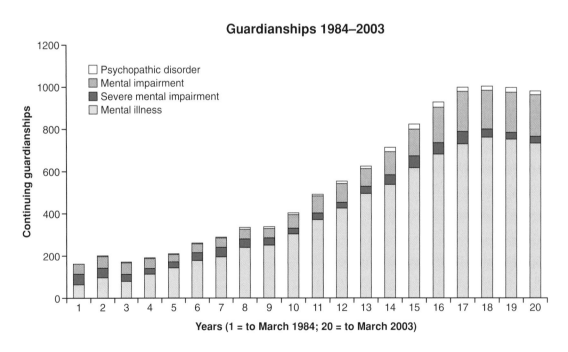

FIGURE 4.1 Guardianships 1984–2003 (Data from Department of Health (2003). *Guardianship Under the Mental Health Act 1983*. London: Department of Health.)

on a given date, the numbers have stabilized as people tend to stay in guardianship for longer periods. On 31 March 2003, there were 975 people in guardianship compared with 161 in 1984. Figure 4.1 illustrates this increased use of guardianship. The introduction of supervised aftercare meant that people paid more attention to guardianship, and this may have contributed to the acceleration in its use.

Purpose

According to the Code of Practice, Paragraph 13.1:

> The purpose of guardianship is to enable patients to receive care in the community where it cannot be provided without the use of compulsory powers. It provides an authoritative framework for working with a patient, with a minimum of constraint, to achieve as independent a life as possible within the community. Where it is used it must be part of the patient's overall care and treatment plan.

Routes and comparison with the Mental Health Act 1959

Guardianship is possible through:

- a civil route: Section 7 of the Mental Health Act – application for guardianship;
- the courts: Section 37 of the Mental Health Act – powers of courts to order hospital admission or guardianship.

The guardian may be either the local authority or a private individual approved by the local authority. In 2002, there were 1012 cases where the local authority was the guardian and only 12 cases where the guardian was a private individual.

In either case, the guardian has certain essential powers to enable them to provide for the patient's care. These are very similar to those of supervised aftercare and are set out below. They involve requirements to reside in a particular place, to attend places for treatment, etc., and to allow greater access to the patient by relevant professionals. These limited powers are in stark contrast to the Mental Health Act 1959, where the guardian had powers equivalent to those of the parent of a child under the age of 14 years. It was believed (probably erroneously) that the powers were seen as too great and that to reduce them would encourage the use of guardianship.

Apart from the reduction from general to specific powers, there is one other major change compared with the earlier Act; with hindsight, this seems like a mistake. The change from 'subnormality' to 'mental impairment' drastically reduced the use of guardianship for people with learning difficulties. Although guardianship is often seen as having a strong protective function, many people who might benefit from this are excluded from guardianship as a result of the new definition of mental impairment, i.e. requiring association with abnormal aggression or seriously irresponsible conduct.

By way of contrast, the inclusion of dementia within the classification of mental illness has led to a dramatic increase in the use of guardianship in this group.

Comparison with the previous Code of Practice

The previous Code of Practice was frequently (mis)quoted as being generally against the use of guardianship. For example, the following statement was often quoted out of context:

> [It] should never be used solely for the purpose of transferring an unwilling person into residential care.

The important word here was 'solely', but as the sentence was not found helpful it has now been deleted.

Paragraph 13.10 of the Code of Practice states:

> Where an adult is assessed as requiring residential care but owing to mental incapacity is unable to make a decision as to whether he or she wishes to be placed in residential care, those who are responsible for his or her care should consider the applicability and appropriateness of guardianship for providing the framework within which decisions about his or her current and future care can be planned.

The revisions to the Code of Practice, introduced in 1999, also contain new advice on the degree of cooperation needed, i.e. '*depending on the patient's level of "capacity"* his or her recognition of the authority of and willingness to work with the guardian' are needed. 'The guardian should be willing to advocate on behalf of the patient in relation to those agencies whose services are needed to carry out the care plan' (revisions in italics).

Grounds

First, nobody under the age of 16 years can be received or placed in guardianship. For a mentally disordered child under the age of 16 who requires some supervision in the community, childcare law (including the rights of parents and the local authority) is available.

The grounds for guardianship under Section 7 or Section 37 are very similar. Here we concentrate on the more common civil route (check Section 37 if necessary).

Section 7(2) of the Mental Health Act 1983 states:

> A guardianship application may be made in respect of a patient on the grounds that
>
> (a) he is suffering from mental disorder, being mental illness, severe mental impairment, psychopathic disorder or mental impairment and his mental disorder is of a nature or degree which warrants his reception into guardianship under this section; and
> (b) it is necessary in the interests of the welfare of the patient or for the protection of other persons that the patient should be so received.

Note that the mental disorder must be one of the four specific classifications, as with a detention for treatment under Section 3, i.e.

- mental illness
- severe mental impairment
- mental impairment
- psychopathic disorder.

This means that 'arrested or incomplete development of mind' is not sufficient and must be associated with abnormally aggressive or seriously irresponsible conduct, thus becoming mental impairment.

Application

The applicant may be an approved social worker or the nearest relative, as defined in Section 26.

The application is based on two medical recommendations and is made to the local authority. Social services departments vary in their procedures for making decisions on guardianship applications; some are explicit in their attitude to this piece of legislation, either being against its use or encouraging it. The relevant local authority is the one where the patient lives, unless the guardian is a private individual, in which case their address determines the relevant authority.

Powers of the guardian

The guardian's powers are set out in Section 8(1). They give the guardian:

- the power to require the patient to reside at a place specified by the authority or the person named as guardian;
- the power to require the patient to attend at places and times so specified for the purpose of medical treatment, occupation, education or training;
- the power to require access to the patient to be given, at any place where the patient is residing, to any medical practitioner, approved social worker or other person so specified.

Paragraph 40 of the Memorandum to the 1983 Act suggests that:

- the power to require the patient to reside at a place specified by the authority or person named as guardian 'may be used to discourage the patient from sleeping rough or living with people who may exploit or mistreat him, or to ensure that he resides in a particular hostel or other facility';
- the places the patient may be required to attend for the purpose of medical treatment, occupation, education or training could 'include a local authority day centre, or a hospital, surgery or clinic';
- the power to require access to the patient to be given, at any place where the patient is residing, to any medical practitioner, approved social worker or other person so specified 'could be used, for example, to ensure that the patient did not neglect himself'.

The powers are essentially the same as those for supervised aftercare, but there is no power to convey, except where the person has absconded from the place of residence.

Consent to treatment

Note that Part IV of the Act on consent to treatment does not apply to guardianship. Thus, there is no statutory route to make a patient accept treatment, such as medication, against his or her will.

Court of Protection

As guardianship does not give any powers in relation to property and affairs, it sometimes goes hand in hand with the use of the Court of Protection.

Time limits

Guardianship lasts for up to six months. It is then renewable for a further six months, and yearly thereafter.

SUPERVISED AFTERCARE (SUPERVISED DISCHARGE)

Three amendments to the Act commenced in 1996. Changes concerning leave of absence and patients absent without leave are dealt with elsewhere. The main changes concerned supervised aftercare, dealt with here. Public reaction to apparent examples of a breakdown in community-care arrangements (e.g. Christopher Clunis, Ben Silcock, see Chapter 1) plus concern with 'revolving-door patients' led to the introduction of this measure. The government considered that a small group of patients needed closer supervision than was available. The measure was linked to the care-programme approach (CPA) and Section 117 aftercare. There were 187 new supervised aftercare cases in England when it was first used in 1996–97, 318 in 1997–98 and 445 in 1998–99. Most National Health Service (NHS) Trusts had just two or three new cases in 1998–99, but a few used it more frequently (e.g. Bolton had 16 new cases, South Tees 15, West Hertfordshire 11 and South West London 15).

Supervised aftercare was seen primarily as a health measure. It looks like guardianship (with additional powers to convey, and driven by health rather than social services), but the government saw it as separate and targeting a different group of patients. It is interesting to note, despite the emphasis on it being a health-led measure, with community psychiatric nurses seen as the most likely supervisors, that in Scotland the role is taken on by a social worker, a mental health officer (equivalent to an approved social worker in England and Wales). Comparisons between the two systems are interesting.

Purpose

The aims of supervised aftercare are to:

- ensure that the patient receives Section 117 aftercare services when they leave hospital;
- provide formal supervision after discharge.

Patients to whom it applies

The patient must be at least 16 years old and already be liable to be detained under one of the following sections:

- Section 3: admission for treatment;
- Section 37: hospital order (made by a magistrates' or crown court);
- Section 47: transfer direction of sentenced prisoner (made by the Home Secretary, without restrictions);
- Section 48: transfer direction of prisoners who have not been sentenced (made by the Home Secretary, without restrictions).

Note that:

- the patient could be on Section 17 leave when Section 25A is applied for and accepted;
- the patient could agree to stay on in hospital, informally, for a period before leaving, and the application would then take effect when he or she leaves hospital.

Grounds

The grounds for supervised aftercare are that:

- the patient is suffering from a specific mental disorder (as for Section 3);
- there would be a substantial risk of serious harm to the health or safety of the patient, or the safety of other people, or of the patient being seriously exploited if he or she was not to receive Section 117 aftercare;
- being subject to aftercare under supervision is likely to help ensure that the patient receives such services.

Applicants

The following are involved in the process of applying for supervised aftercare for a patient:

- The responsible medical officer (RMO) makes the application on form 1S.
- The application is addressed to the relevant health authority.
- The health authority must consult with the relevant social services department.
- Recommendations are needed from a doctor (form 2S) and from an approved social worker (form 3S).

- Signatures are needed from both the proposed community responsible medical officer (CRMO) and the proposed supervisor to indicate that they will take on the role.

Further details of the processes involved are given below.

Effects

There will be:

- a CRMO;
- a supervisor (e.g. a community psychiatric nurse or social worker);
- a record of any planned aftercare services and any requirements placed on the individual.

Length

The supervised aftercare lasts for six months. It is renewable once for six months and annually thereafter. The patient and his or her nearest relative can appeal to the Mental Health Review Tribunal once in each period.

Powers conferred

Under Section 25D, the aftercare bodies may impose any of the following requirements:

(a) that the patient reside at a specified place;
(b) that the patient attend at specified places and times for the purpose of medical treatment, occupation, education or training; and
(c) that access to the patient be given, at any place where the patient is residing, to the supervisor, any registered medical practitioner or any ASW [approved social worker] or to any other person authorised by the supervisor.

Notes

- The power to take and convey exists for points (a) and (b) above when they are made requirements.
- A patient is not covered by Part IV of the Act, so consent to treatment provisions do not apply and the patient cannot be made to take medication unwillingly.

What the patient must be told if subject to supervised aftercare

Where the health authority accepts a supervision application, the authority must inform the patient, both orally and in writing:

- that the application has been accepted;
- of its effects on the patient;
- of his or her right to appeal to the Mental Health Review Tribunal.

Modification of the aftercare requirements

The aftercare requirements can be modified. Before or after discharge from hospital, the responsible aftercare bodies can review and, if appropriate, modify the services or the requirements. The patient, carer and nearest relative (where appropriate) must be consulted. If the review is because the patient refuses or neglects to receive any of the aftercare services provided, or to comply with any of the specified requirements, then there must be a review of whether supervised aftercare is still needed and whether admission for treatment might be necessary. In the latter case, an approved social worker must be informed. Any compulsory admission then requires new medical recommendations and an application.

Termination

Supervised aftercare may end in any of the following ways:

- The CRMO can end supervised aftercare at any time but must consult with the patient, the supervisor and certain other people before doing so (Section 25H).
- It ends automatically if the patient is detained under Section 3 or is accepted into guardianship.
- The Mental Health Review Tribunal can discharge the patient from supervised aftercare on application from the patient or the nearest relative or reference from the Secretary of State.

Section 117 aftercare

When supervised aftercare ends, Section 117 aftercare does not necessarily end. Health and social services authorities have to agree that a person is no longer in need of such services before the obligation to provide them ends.

Detention under Section 2

If a patient subject to supervised aftercare is detained under Section 2, then the supervised aftercare is suspended. It resumes when the patient is back in the community.

Custody

If a patient subject to supervised aftercare is taken into custody, then the supervised aftercare is suspended. It resumes when the patient is back in the community.

Power to convey

Under Section 25D of the Mental Health Act 1983, a supervisor has the power to convey a patient to a place where they are required to reside or attend only *where these requirements have been specified on the application.*

Guidance on supervised aftercare

This guidance is provided by HSG(96)11/LAC(96)8:

- Advises interagency protocol to cover when power to convey may be used.
- The supervisor may decide to use the power if a patient has got into a situation that is putting him or her, or other people, at risk and needs to be taken home urgently.
- The supervisor may also wish to consider using the power if the patient is not attending for medical treatment and it is thought that this might be overcome by taking him or her to the place where treatment is to be given.
- The supervisor should consider whether problems could be overcome by adjustment to the package of services or if an assessment for re-admission might be necessary.
- The supervisor may authorize any responsible adult to convey. It will normally be advisable to use the ambulance service or, possibly, the police.
- The reasons for use of the power must always be recorded.

Procedure for obtaining supervised aftercare

1   The RMO considers the application and ensures that the following are consulted:

- the patient*;
- one or more members of the hospital-based team;
- one or more professionals who will be concerned with the aftercare services;
- informal carer* (not a professional) who the RMO thinks will play a substantial part in providing the care;
- nearest relative* (unless the patient objects and is not overruled), if practicable.

By involving social services representatives in the above process, this should link with the health authority's requirement to consult with the social services department about a Section 117 plan. A statement of aftercare services to be provided is needed and should be attached to the application.

---

*Paragraph 26 of the Health Service Guidelines/Local Authority Circular HSG/LAC guidance states that these individuals should be 'consulted in a suitable and sensitive manner', with interpreters as needed. It warns of misunderstandings from assumptions based on, for example, gender, social background, ethnic origin, sexual orientation, religion and deafness. Note that the wording of the Act does not require the RMO personally to undertake the consultations, so others could carry this out and feed back to the RMO.

2 The application is normally submitted to the health provider unit. The application must include the names of the CRMO and the supervisor as well as the nearest relative and the informal carer, if consulted. The application should be accompanied by:

- two recommendations, from an approved social worker and a doctor (these should try to see the patient together, or at least within a week of each other; they should also examine records of detention and treatment and the plans for aftercare);
- signed statements from the CRMO and the supervisor that they are willing to act as such;
- statement of aftercare services (in a care plan);
- details of requirements to be imposed on the patient.

Joint protocols on supervised aftercare

The HSG/LAC guidance (Paragraph 9) recommends that health authorities and local authorities should develop local protocols. Annexe C of the HSG(96)11/LAC(96)8 (also known as the Supplement to the Code of Practice) suggests such interagency agreements should cover the following:

- *Shared understanding needed on:*
  - risk-assessment procedure;
  - consultation procedures between the health authority or provider unit and the local authority for consideration of Section 25A, completion of documentation and acceptance of application;
  - reviewing and monitoring;
  - role of supervisor and experience required;
  - power to convey: when to use or not use records, who is authorized, involving ambulance and police services;
  - appeals and complaints.

- *Making the procedure work:*
  - how to provide advocacy and interpretation;
  - which joint procedures to use if the patient does not attend for treatment;
  - integration of CPA, care management and Section 25A;
  - information technology (IT) systems to integrate CPA with supervision registers;
  - performance standards;
  - involvement of users and carers.

- *Implementation planning:*
  - training for supervisors and other professionals;
  - aftercare arrangements discussed with probation, housing, police and general practitioners (GPs).

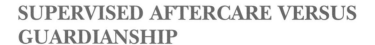

SUPERVISED AFTERCARE VERSUS GUARDIANSHIP

HSG/LAC guidance

Paragraph 8 notes that guardianship remains available as an option but considers that for patients who meet requirements for supervised discharge the latter:

> has advantages: in the specific legal provision it offers for making and reviewing aftercare arrangements and the roles assigned to the community responsible medical officer and supervisor.

Where the grounds for supervised discharge are not met fully, the guidance states that guardianship may well be considered.

COMPARISON OF SUPERVISED AFTERCARE WITH GUARDIANSHIP

Supervised aftercare (Section 25A) is compared with guardianship (Section 7) in Table 4.1.

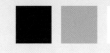
TABLE 4.1 Comparison of supervised aftercare with guardianship

	Aftercare under supervision	Guardianship
Existing status	Aged at least 16 years and liable to detention on sections 3, 37, 47 or 48	Aged at least 16 years
Mental disorder	Mental illness	Mental illness
	Severe mental impairment	Severe mental impairment
	Mental impairment	Mental impairment
	Psychopathic disorder	Psychopathic disorder
Risk level	There would be a substantial risk of serious harm to health or safety of patient, safety of others, or of serious exploitation of patient if not to receive Section 117 aftercare	Necessary in the interests of the welfare of the patient or for the protection of others
Application	RMO	Approved social worker or nearest relative
Recommendations	Approved social worker and doctor	Two doctors
Who accepts?	Health authority	Local authority
Duration	6 months, 6 months, yearly	6 months, 6 months, yearly
Mental Health Review Tribunal	Patient or nearest relative (where informed) can apply	Patient can apply
Who can discharge?	CRMO and MHRT	RMO, MHRT and nearest relative or local authority
When does it end automatically?	If detained on Section 3 or placed in guardianship	If detained on Section 3
Requirements	Reside where specified	Reside where specified
	Attend for treatment, etc.	Attend for treatment, etc.
	Access as authorized	Access as authorized
Power to convey?	Yes (where requirement made for residence and/or attendance)	Not in first instance, but power to return to required place of residence
Part IV Consent to Treatment rules?	Not covered by Part IV	Not covered by Part IV
Will Section 117 aftercare apply?	Yes	Only if patient previously on section 3, 37, 47 or 48
Covered by CPA	Yes	Yes

CPA, care-programme approach; CRMO, community responsible medical officer; MHRT, Mental Health Review Tribunal; RMO, responsible medical officer.

5

Patients concerned in criminal proceedings or under sentence

In this chapter, the following topics will be considered:

- detention at a police station
- court procedure
- disposal/sentencing.

Ultimately, nowadays, the aim of the criminal justice system is to try to divert away from the court system as many mentally disordered people as possible.

CRIMINAL RESPONSIBILITY

Criminal responsibility is a legal concept that begins at the age of ten years in England and Wales and eight years in Scotland (*doli incapax*). It is questionable how good psychiatrists are in judging responsibility as opposed to diagnosing mental disorder.

Most offences require some form of intent (*mens rea*) as well as an unlawful act (*actus reus*). These offences are divided into those that require specific intent, such as murder, rape and arson, and those that require only basic intent. Some minor offences, such as motoring offences, do not require *mens rea*. Certain mental states interfere with the defendant's (patient's) intent and may give rise to defences in law to the offences.

Insanity has always been regarded as a defence in English law. For example, as mentioned in Chapter 1, a judge in King Alfred's time was hanged for having ordered the hanging of an insane man. By the early eighteenth century, for insanity to be a defence in law it had to be such as to cause the subject to be 'like a wild beast', devoid of all reason and memory. However, in 1780, a soldier was acquitted of murder because he was found to be suffering from a delusion about the victim as a result of insanity.

MENTALLY DISORDERED OFFENDERS INVOLVED WITH THE POLICE AND COURTS

Following an arrest, an individual may be:

- admitted informally to a psychiatric hospital; *or*
- detained compulsorily under civil sections of the Mental Health Act 1983 (e.g. section 2, 3, 4 or 136); *and/or*
- cautioned by the police, so long as the individual accepts his or her guilt; *or*
- charged and taken to court (either on or not on bail).

In any event, the police will check to determine whether the person is an absconding patient; if so, the police will return the patient to hospital under section 18 or 138.

Under the **Police and Criminal Evidence Act 1984** (PACE), there is a code of practice that covers the detention, treatment and questioning of a person by a police officer. If the individual is suspected by a police officer to be mentally disordered, then an 'appropriate adult' must be informed and asked to go to the police station. This person ideally should be an individual trained or experienced in dealing with mentally disordered people, rather than an unqualified relative. An appropriate adult should be present while the individual is told their rights and can advise the person being interviewed, observe the fairness of the interview, and facilitate communication with the interviewee. They may also require the presence of a lawyer.

If a decision is taken by the police to prosecute, then the case is passed to the Crown Prosecution Service, which will also consider the public interest and the likely adverse effects of prosecution of a mentally disordered individual.

Court procedure

The presumption is always in favour of remanding an individual on bail rather than in custody. Bail could include a condition of residence in a psychiatric hospital, although the individual would be an informal patient there unless otherwise detained under the Mental Health Act 1983.

Where a person might otherwise be remanded to prison, the Mental Health Act 1983 allows for the following three possibilities:

- remand to hospital for a report, under Section 35;
- remand to hospital for treatment, under Section 36;
- remand to hospital of other prisoners (including those on remand in custody), under Section 48.

At many Magistrates' Courts there are diversion teams in attendance on certain days. These teams are made up of a psychiatrist plus a community psychiatric nurse (CPN) and social worker and are there to assess mentally disordered defendants. The benefit of these teams is that they allow defendants in custody to be assessed quickly and diverted into the mental health system if appropriate. The scheme also allows for the courts and prosecution to be appraised of a defendant's condition more quickly than may be the case otherwise.

Section 35: remand to hospital for report

This order can be made under Subsection (3)

> (a) if the court is satisfied on the written or oral evidence of a registered medical practitioner that there is reason to suspect the accused person is suffering from mental illness, psychopathic disorder, severe mental impairment or mental impairment; and (b) the court is of the opinion that it would be impractical for a report on his mental condition to be made if he were remanded on bail.

A hospital bed must be available within seven days. If awaiting a bed, the accused must be kept in a 'place of safety', e.g. 'police station, prison or remand centre or any hospital the managers of which are willing temporarily to receive him' (Section 55(1)).

The remand is for a maximum period of 28 days, although it is renewable for further periods of 28 days, without the necessity of the patient attending court, up to a maximum of 12 weeks. Part IV provisions on consent to treatment do not apply, so an individual cannot be treated without his or her consent, except in an emergency under common law. Some psychiatrists additionally detain such individuals under Section 3 if they wish to treat them without their consent; the Code of Practice states that this may be considered if there is a delay in getting to court. The use of Section 36 might, however, then be more appropriate.

Section 36: remand to hospital for treatment

This may be used only by the Crown Court and is an alternative to remand to custody. It can apply to those waiting for trial or sentence. It requires the written or oral evidence of two doctors that the individual is 'suffering from mental illness or severe mental impairment (only) of a nature or degree which makes it appropriate for him to be detained in hospital for treatment'. It cannot be used for a person charged with murder.

The remand is for a maximum of 28 days, although this may be renewed for further periods of 28 days, without the necessity of the patient attending court, up to a maximum of 12 weeks. Part IV provisions of consent to treatment apply.

A hospital bed must be available within seven days; the individual must meanwhile be kept in a 'place of safety' (Section 55(1)).

Problems arise if an individual has to wait for more than the maximum 12 weeks of the order to appear in the Crown Court. In these circumstances, detention under a civil section or the use of Section 48 may be required.

Section 48: transfer direction to hospital for remanded criminal and sentenced civil prisoners

This section gives the Home Secretary powers to direct the transfer to hospital of a person waiting for trial or sentence and who has been remanded in custody. It also applies to people detained under the Immigration Act 1971 and sentenced civil prisoners.

The Home Secretary requires two medical reports, which do not need to specify the availability of a bed at a particular hospital, stating that a person is suffering from mental illness or severe mental impairment of a nature or degree that makes it appropriate for him or her to be detained in hospital for medical treatment and that he or she is in urgent need of such treatment.

The period of detention is variable and can continue to the time of sentence. A Section 49 restriction direction may be added by the Home Office (pg 53, Table 5.1). Section 48 has been used increasingly to divert severely mentally ill (psychotic) offenders from custody to hospital, even when the need may not be 'urgent'. It has the advantage that it does not require a court hearing to impose the order. On occasions, for instance when an acutely mentally ill offender has appeared in court, such an individual may be remanded only nominally to a named custodial facility and, by arrangement with the Home Office, is transferred directly to hospital without being placed in custody.

MENTAL ABNORMALITY AS A DEFENCE IN COURT

In some cases, a person charged with an offence offers evidence of his or her mental disturbance either:

(a) to excuse his being tried (not fit to plead), or
(b) to agree to having done the act but not to have been fully responsible at the time (insane or diminished responsibility or automatism or infanticide).

Thus, in these cases, the psychiatric evidence is presented as part of the arguments to the court and is heard before conviction.

Unfit to plead: Criminal Procedure (Insanity and Unfitness to Plead) Act 1991

A mentally disordered defendant may assert that he or she is unfit to plead (under 'disability' in relation to trial). This refers to the time of trial. The defendant would have to prove, using medical evidence, in a Crown Court hearing that he or she was not fit to do at least one of the following (based on the original test used in *R* v. *Pritchard* (1836)):

■ instruct counsel ('so as to make a proper defence');
■ appreciate the significance of pleading;
■ challenge a juror;
■ examine a witness;
■ understand and follow the evidence of court procedure.

Note that the defendant does not have to be fit to give evidence him- or herself.

If it appears that a defendant is unfit to plead but may, in time and with treatment, become fit, then the case is often adjourned to allow for that improvement in the defendant's mental state. If, however, the defendant does not become fit, then the unfitness to plead procedure will have to be followed. If raised by the judge or the prosecution, this must be proved beyond reasonable doubt; but if raised by the defence, this has to be proved only on the balance of probabilities. This is a very rare plea and is likely to be successful only in cases such as severe mental impairment or for patients who are extremely paranoid, e.g. about the court or their legal representatives. Physical illness, e.g. pneumonia, may also result in unfitness to plead and stand trial.

The procedure requires that first there is a trial (with a jury) to determine whether the defendant is fit to plead. The jury will have to hear evidence (written or oral) from at least two Section 12 Mental Health Act 1983-approved doctors before reaching their decision. If the jury finds that a defendant is fit to plead, then the defendant will stand trial as normal in front of a different jury. If a defendant is found unfit to plead, then there is also a second trial, but only to determine whether the defendant committed the act alleged (*actus reus*) and not to consider the defendant's mental state (*mens rea*).

If found unfit to plead and to have committed the act, then a defendant can be sentenced only to a hospital order, guardianship order, supervision and treatment order, or absolute discharge. Historically, this concept originates from dealing with deaf mutes. In medieval times, defendants were pressed under weights to give a plea, without which they could not be convicted or executed or their property given to the Exchequer; hence the phrase 'press for an answer'.

On rare occasions, one may be asked to help the court decide whether an offender who appears to be mute (i.e. there is no speech at all) is being mute by 'malice or by visitation of God'. If mute 'by malice', then the case proceeds with a not guilty plea entered on the defendant's behalf. If mute 'by visitation of God', i.e. deaf and dumb, then the question of fitness to plead will arise with a view to disposal under the Criminal Procedure (Insanity and Unfitness to Plead) Act 1991.

In Scotland, individuals are found unfit to plead more commonly, including in cases where in England they would be convicted and detained under a Section 37 hospital order. Fitness to plead is also often a major issue in the USA, where the term 'competency' is used.

Note that the unfit-to-plead procedure relates only to Crown Court cases; there is no such procedure in a Magistrates' Court. In less serious cases, where there is evidence that the defendant is mentally disordered, then cases can be dealt with in the Magistrates' Court under Section 37(3) of the Mental Health Act 1983. This procedure allows for the facts of an alleged offence (*actus reus*) to be proved so that the court is satisfied that the defendant did the act or made the omission charged, again without regard to the defendant's mental state at the time of the offence. If the defendant is proved to have committed the act, then he or she will be made the subject of a hospital order.

Not guilty by reason of insanity ('special verdict'; insanity defence; McNaughton Rules): Criminal Procedure (Insanity and Unfitness to Plead) Act 1991

Historically, this defence arose from the case of Daniel McNaughton in 1843. McNaughton, believing himself to be poisoned by Whigs, attempted to shoot the

Prime Minister, Robert Peel, missed (or perhaps misidentified), and shot and killed Peel's secretary. Because McNaughton was deluded and insane, he was acquitted, but this caused a great deal of argument, including from Queen Victoria ('Insane he may be, but not guilty he is not'), and the law lords were asked to issue guidance for the courts in response to five questions. Their guidance is known as the McNaughton Rules.

In this defence, the offender is arguing that he or she is not guilty (not deserving of punishment) by reason of his or her insanity. It has to be proved to a court, on the balance of probabilities, that *at the time of the offence*, the offender laboured under such defect of reason that he or she met the McNaughton Rules, i.e.

(1) That by reason of such defect from disease of the mind, he did not know the nature or quality of his act (this means the physical nature of the act), *or*

(2) Not know that what he was doing was wrong (forbidden by law).

(3) If an individual was suffering from a delusion, then his actions would be judged by their relationship to the delusion, i.e. if he believed his life to be immediately threatened, then he would be justified in striking out, but not otherwise.

Technically, this plea may be put forward for any offence, but in practice it is put forward usually only for murder or other serious offences. In fact, such a plea is rare.

Evidence from two or more medical practitioners, one of whom is approved under Section 12 of the Mental Health Act 1983, is required before the return of the verdict not guilty by reason of insanity. Such a verdict implies lack of intent. However, a psychiatrist can give evidence only regarding an individual's capacity to form intent (a legal concept), not the fact of intent at the time of the offence.

Under the Criminal Procedure Act 1991, if the defendant is found not guilty by reason of insanity, the judge has the freedom to decide on the sentencing and disposal of the defendant, i.e. discretionary sentencing, including detention in hospital under forensic treatment orders of the Mental Health Act 1983.

Diminished responsibility

As a reaction against the fact that mentally disordered people who had killed were still being hanged despite the McNaughton Rules, a movement was created to bring in a defence of diminished responsibility, i.e. the responsibility of the offender is not totally absent because of mental abnormality but is only partially impaired; therefore, the offender would be found guilty but the sentence modified. This was made law in the **Homicide Act 1957** and applies only to a charge of murder. The murder charge is reduced to manslaughter on the grounds of diminished responsibility.

Under the 1957 Homicide Act (Section 2), as a defence against the charge (only) of murder, the offender may plead that at the time of the offence, he or she had diminished responsibility. The offender has to show that at the time

where a person kills ... he shall not be convicted of murder if he was suffering from *such abnormality of mind*, whether arising from a condition of arrested or retarded development of mind or any inherent causes or induced by disease or injury, *as substantially impaired his mental responsibility for his acts.*

Abnormality of mind

'Abnormality of mind' is left to the defendant (or his or her medical advisors) to define and is not synonymous with mental disorder as defined in the Mental Health Act 1983. It has been ruled in the Court of Appeal regarding this defence that 'abnormality of mind' would have affected at the time of the offence the individual's perception, judgement (between right and wrong, between good and bad) and/or the voluntary control of (capacity to control, a legal concept) his or her actions. Thus, abnormality of mind is:

> a state of mind so different from that of the ordinary human beings that the reasonable man, earlier defined as 'a man with a normal mind', would term it abnormal. It appears to us to be wide enough to cover the mind's activities in all its aspects, not only the perception of physical acts and matters, and the ability to form a rational judgement as to whether the act was right or wrong, but also the ability to exercise will power to control physical acts in accordance with that rational judgement. (*R* v. *Byrne* (1960))

The authoritative interpretation of the term 'abnormality of mind' was given by Lord Parker (*R* v. *Byrne* (1960)) as follows:

> Whether the accused was at the time of killing suffering from 'any abnormality of mind' in the broad sense in which we have indicated above is a question for the jury. On this question medical evidence is, no doubt, important, but the jury are entitled to take into consideration all the evidence including the acts or statements of the accused and his demeanour. They are not bound to accept the medical evidence, if there is other material before them which, in their good judgement, conflicts with it and outweighs it. The aetiology of the abnormality of mind (namely, whether it arose from a condition of arrested or retarded development of mind or any inherent causes or was induced by disease or injury) does, however, seem to be a matter to be determined on expert evidence ...

Substantially

'Substantially' is also undefined and is left to the jury to decide, although the doctors will have to give their opinions.

> Substantial does not mean total ... At the other end [it] does not mean minimal or trivial. It is something in between. (*R* v. *Lloyd* (1966))

Successful plea

The effect of a successful plea is to reduce the charge from murder to manslaughter. Murder carries a statutory sentence of life imprisonment, but the court is free to make any sentence at all with regard to manslaughter, including a hospital or a community rehabilitation order or, indeed, a life prison sentence, in

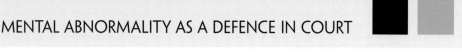

which case research has shown that such individuals may spend longer in custody than those convicted of murder (Dell 1984). The verdict 'unties the judge's hands'. In addition to a report supporting the plea of diminished responsibility, the psychiatrist may also, if appropriate, wish to arrange for the appropriate hospital treatment and offer the appropriate section recommendations to the court to help them with their sentencing.

Use

The diminished responsibility defence has been used where a defence of insanity would have no hope of success. Examples include:

- mercy killing;
- when the subject kills his or her spouse in a state of reactive depression;
- individuals who kill in jealous frenzies;
- individuals who are subject to an 'irresistible impulse' to kill (cited more often in the USA);
- subjects who kill and who are 'deranged' by psychopathic disorder.

The diminished responsibility defence has largely replaced the insanity defence. There are about 200 cases per year in England and Wales; less than half of these get a hospital order.

Retrospective mental state assessment

The psychiatrist carries out a retrospective mental state examination for the time of the offence when assessing whether the defendant is not guilty by reason of insanity (McNaughton Rules) or whether diminished responsibility applies. In the McNaughton Rules, the legal concept used is *disease of mind*. In diminished responsibility, the legal concept used is *abnormality of mind*. From case law:

- mind = reason, memory, understanding;
- disease = organic/functional, permanent/temporary, treatable/not treatable, is 'internal' (*R* v. *Quick* (1973)) and/or 'manifests in violence and is prone to recur' (*Bratty* v. *A. G.* in Northern Ireland (1961)). It also includes epilepsy (*R* v. *Sullivan* (1983)).

Criticism of McNaughton Rules and diminished responsibility

McNaughton Rules

These rules are now almost obsolete. Points against them include the following:

- Hardly anybody is mad enough to fit the rules (Lord Bramwell). Even McNaughton would not have been.
- The rules assume a doctrine that mind is made up of separate independent compartments, of which cognition is most important (a Victorian view).
- The rules are too unfair, as abnormal mental states do not fit into rigid categories.
- The rules ignore the importance of emotional disturbance and failure of will when cognition is normal.

Diminished responsibility

The most important points in favour of this are that:

- it allows for an overall assessment of the person;
- it leads to more flexible sentencing.

Against diminished responsibility are the following points:

- There is a problem of balancing the concept of responsibility with 'determinism', e.g. does a greater propensity to lose one's temper imply less responsibility?
- It assumes that a distinction can be made between psychopathy and wickedness in terms of moral or criminal responsibility.
- Does diminished responsibility mean less power to resist temptation? If so, should the irresponsible be punished less than the responsible?
- Does an irresponsible act in a normally responsible person indicate a greater aberration of mind than irresponsible behaviour in the irresponsible?
- If a person is found to have diminished responsibility, then it may mean that the court will return such a person to society faster than a responsible offender.

In fact, those who are given a custodial sentence following a successful plea of diminished responsibility (Dell 1984) spend longer in custody than those convicted of murder, who serve a mean of 11.5 years before being released on life licence. This may reflect concern that while abnormality of mind was identified in these cases of diminished responsibility, no ameliorating treatment of it was undertaken, for example in hospital, if the individual received a life prison sentence.

Automatism

This is a rare plea generally restricted (though not entirely) to cases of homicide. The defendant pleads that at the time of the offence, his or her behaviour was automatic (no *mens rea*). The law uses this term to mean a state almost near unconsciousness. It refers to unconscious, involuntary, non-purposeful acts where the mind is not conscious of what the body is doing. There is a separation between the will and the act, or the mind and the act ('Mind does not go with what is being done' (*Bratty* v. *A. G.* in Northern Ireland (1961))).

Automatism has been pleaded successfully, particularly in cases of homicide, for offences occurring during hypoglycaemic attacks, sleepwalking and sleep, e.g. fighting tigers and snakes in dreams (theoretically, this should be during night terrors in slow-wave sleep, since during dreams involving complex visual images, one should be paralysed in rapid-eye-movement (REM) sleep, but it has been argued that such offences may occur as an individual wakes from a dream). Such must be the degree of automatism that there is no capacity to form any intent to kill or any capacity to control actions.

In certain cases, e.g. offending while sleepwalking, the accused has walked free from the court on the understanding that he or she will always lock their bedroom door when sleeping.

Where a defence of non-insane automatism is put forward, the subject is hoping to receive a total acquittal. However, the law has become aware that some automatism states are really the result, in the legal sense, of a disease of the mind, e.g. epilepsy, that may recur. Therefore, in such cases, the jury may be invited to consider that the defence of automatism should be regarded as evidence of insanity (*insane automatism*) and to return a special verdict of 'not guilty by reason of insanity', which would allow for discretionary sentencing, including detention in hospital.

While, historically, sleepwalking and night terrors have been accepted as automatisms and have led to acquittal, case law (Lord Justice Lawton) now differentiates *non-insane automatism due to external causes*, e.g. hypoglycaemia caused by insulin, from *insane automatism due to disease of the mind caused by mental illness or brain disease (intrinsic factors)*, e.g. diabetes, epilepsy and even hysterical dissociative fugue states, in which a special verdict of not guilty by reason of insanity should be returned.

HOMICIDE

Definition

Homicide is the killing of another human being. It is not necessarily unlawful.

Epidemiology

In 1996, there were 627 homicides in England and Wales; of these, 161 were manslaughter and 78 were diminished responsibility. Two hundred and seventeen of the victims were female (half were killed by their partners). This compares with 16 000 externally caused deaths (of these, half were suicides, others misadventure, accidents, etc.).

Legal classification

Homicide may be lawful or unlawful.

Lawful homicide

Lawful homicide may be:

- justifiable, e.g. on behalf of the state, such as actions taken by people in the army or the police;
- excusable, e.g. a pure accident or an honest or reasonable mistake.

Unlawful homicide

Unlawful homicide is the unlawful killing of any reasonable creature in being and under the Queen's (or King's) Peace. Types of unlawful homicide include:

- murder
- manslaughter
- child destruction
- genocide
- causing death by dangerous driving
- suicide pacts
- infanticide.

Some of these are considered further here.

Murder

Murder is an offence at common law. It is defined as an unlawful killing with *malice aforethought*. Malice aforethought requires either an intention to kill or cause grievous bodily harm. Murder, like any other crime requiring proof of intent, involves proof of a subjective state of mind on the part of the accused. The *actus reus* of murder consists of both of the following:

- an unlawful act;
- the act causes the death of another human being.

Murder results in a mandatory life sentence. In England and Wales, an average of 11.5 years is served in prison, and then the prisoner is released on life licence. A few murderers do serve life.

Manslaughter

Manslaughter may be categorized into three groups, namely:

- voluntary manslaughter
- involuntary manslaughter
- corporate liability.

The third of these will not be considered further here.

VOLUNTARY MANSLAUGHTER

These are cases of homicide in which the defendant would be guilty of murder if it were not for the availability of one of the following partial defences:

- Diminished responsibility (Section 2 Homicide Act 1957).
- Provocation (Section 3 Homicide Act 1957): it is considered to be sudden or temporary loss of control under provocation that might make a normal person kill. Whether this occurred is for the jury to decide, although a psychiatrist's opinion may be requested. More recently, psychiatric evidence about the propensity of individuals with certain vulnerable personalities or conditions, such as learning disability, to be provoked has been accepted as admissible.
- Killing in pursuance of a suicide pact (which the offender has to prove) (Section 4 Homicide Act 1957): a suicide pact is defined as being a common agreement between two or more persons, having for its object the death of all of them, whether or not each is to take his or her own life.

INVOLUNTARY MANSLAUGHTER

Involuntary manslaughter refers to cases of homicide without malice aforethought. It can take several forms, including:

- an unlawful and dangerous act – 'constructive manslaughter': the *actus reus* consists of an unlawful act that is dangerous and causes death;
- gross negligence: the *actus reus* consists of a breach of a duty of care that the accused owes to the victim, with the result that this breach leads to the victim's death.

Infanticide

Under the **Infanticide Acts 1922 and 1938** (Section 1), infanticide is defined as having occurred when a woman by any wilful act caused the death of her child under the age of 12 months, but at the time of the act or omission the balance of her mind was 'disturbed by reason of her not being fully recovered from the effect of giving birth to the child or the effect of lactation consequent upon the birth of the child'. This is technically an offence rather than a defence.

The grounds for this plea, as an alternative to murder, are less stringent than those for diminished responsibility (i.e. there is no need to prove abnormality of mind); nor do they require proof of a mental disorder, e.g. mental illness. It is the policy of the Director of Public Prosecution and the Crown Prosecution Service to use this plea for such mothers. It does not apply to adopted children or to any child other than the youngest (otherwise a manslaughter plea has to be used), as it is possible to give birth to two children within one year.

When this plea was introduced, many such mothers had acute organic confusional puerperal psychoses. Nowadays, infanticide is rather an historical anachronism: only about one in six of such mothers have functional puerperal psychoses, the remainder being not dissimilar from those who batter their children. It usually results in a sentence of a community rehabilitation order, often with a condition of psychiatric treatment (outpatient or inpatient).

AMNESIA

Amnesia is not in itself a defence; the underlying condition may, for example, be a post-traumatic state, epileptic fits or acute psychosis. In the 1959 Podola Appeal case (Podola's amnesia was, in fact, not genuine), it was ruled that even if amnesia is genuine, it is no bar to trial.

Amnesia may be feigned by lying or caused by:

- hysterical amnesia (denial)
- failure of registration owing to overarousal
- alcohol
- other psychoactive drugs
- head injury.

Between 40 and 50 per cent of people charged with homicide claim amnesia for the actual act.

DRUGS AND ALCOHOL

It has always been considered that a person is fully responsible for their actions if they knowingly used drugs or alcohol (voluntary intoxication). It is assumed that everyone knows that drunkenness is associated with aggressive and irresponsible behaviour and therefore one is responsible for not becoming drunk. The same rule applies to drug abuse. This would not apply if an individual were 'slipped' drugs or alcohol, or if their doctor did not inform them of side effects and interactions (e.g. with alcohol) of medication, e.g. benzodiazepines, which, in particular, have been cited by shoplifters as a defence for, although almost never the cause of, shoplifting. Such issues may also arise following the consumption of over-the-counter medications such as cold cures and nose drops, which may contain, for instance, ephedrine.

Successful defences have been based on:

- being so drunk as to be incapable of forming intent in offences requiring specific intent;
- developing a mental illness, e.g. psychosis, as a result of the ingestion of a drug or alcohol (as in delirium tremens), and acting under the influence of such a mental illness, which may allow the defence of not guilty by reason of insanity or diminished responsibility;
- where the use of a drug, which might be quite legitimate, produces a mental state abnormality that could not have been anticipated by the subject, e.g. hypoglycaemia after the use of insulin. For such an abnormal mental state to be used successfully as a defence, it must be shown that the accused took reasonable precautions (e.g. in the case of insulin, not to become hypoglycaemic), and yet these precautions failed. In one case, a man who had drunk 12 pints of beer before an offence cited, successfully, the effect of consuming a large amount of fluid, rather than the alcohol, as the precipitating cause of his mental state. It was demonstrated that his electroencephalographic recording became disturbed when he drank 12 pints of water, and it was argued that the fluid itself, and not the alcohol, had been the cause of his abnormality.

Thus, overall, successful defences following consumption of alcohol or drugs are based on either (i) involuntary intoxication or (ii) if intoxicated voluntarily, lack of specific intent where offences require this.

Note that the term 'pathological intoxication' (used in the *International Statistical Classification of Diseases and Related Health Problems*, 10th revision (ICD-10)) refers to a sudden onset of aggression and often violent behaviour, not typical of an individual when sober, very soon after drinking amounts of alcohol (only) that would not produce intoxication in most people.

SENTENCING

The following sentences available under the Mental Health Act 1983 are detailed in Table 5.1:

- hospital order: Section 37;
- interim hospital order: Section 38;
- restriction order: Section 41;
- guardianship order: Section 37;
- hospital and limitation directions: Section 45A.

TABLE 5.1 Forensic treatment orders for mentally abnormal offenders

	Grounds	Made by	Medical recommendation	Maximum duration	Eligibility for appeal to Mental Health Review Tribunal
Section 35: remand to hospital for report	Mental disorder	Magistrates' or Crown Court	Any doctor	28 days Renewable at 28-day intervals Maximum 12 weeks	–
Section 36: remand to hospital for treatment	Mental illness Severe mental impairment (not if charged with murder)	Crown Court	Two doctors: one approved under Section 12	28 days Renewable at 28-day intervals Maximum 12 weeks	–
Section 37 (hospital and guardianship orders) N.B. (Section 37 [3] without conviction)	Mental disorder (if psychopathic disorder or mental impairment, must be likely to alleviate or prevent deterioration) Accused or convicted of an imprisonable offence	Magistrates' or Crown Court	Two doctors: one approved under Section 12	6 months Renewable for further 6 months and then annually	During second 6 months Then every year Mandatory every 3 years
Section 41: restriction order	Added to Section 37 to protect public from serious harm	Crown Court	Oral evidence from one doctor	Usually without limit of time Effect: leave, transfer or discharge only with consent from Home Secretary	As for Section 37
Section 38: interim hospital order	Mental disorder For trial of treatment	Magistrates' or Crown Court	Two doctors: one approved under Section 12	12 weeks Renewable at 28-day intervals Maximum 12 months	None
Section 47: transfer of sentenced prisoner to hospital	Mental disorder	Home Secretary	Two doctors: one approved under Section 12	Until earliest date of release (EDR) from sentence	Once in the first 6 months Then once in the next 6 months Thereafter, once a year
Section 48: urgent transfer to hospital of remand prisoner	Mental disorder	Home Secretary	Two doctors: one approved under Section 12	Until date of trial or sentence	Once in the first 6 months Then once in the next 6 months Thereafter, once a year
Section 49: restriction direction	Added to section 47 or 48	Home Secretary	–	Until end of section 47 or 48 Effect: leave, transfer or discharge only with consent of Home Secretary	As for sections 47 and 48

In addition, a community rehabilitation order with a condition of psychiatric treatment is available.

Each of these is now considered in turn.

Section 37: hospital order

This may be made by the Crown Court or a Magistrates' Court, the latter being able to make such an order without conviction under Section 37(3) so long as the court is satisfied that the offender committed the act or omission in question. The individual has to be charged with an imprisonable offence, not just any offence.

For this sentence to be made, a hospital bed must be available within 28 days, beginning from the date of the order. The patient, meanwhile, must be kept in a 'place of safety' (Section 55(1)). The availability of a bed within 28 days and the evidence of two registered medical practitioners, at least one of whom is approved under Section 12 of the Mental Health Act 1983, are essential before the court can impose such an order.

Section 38: interim hospital order

If either a Magistrates' or a Crown Court is uncertain that a full Section 37 hospital order is appropriate, then this can be tested out by making an interim order. This can be made for up to 12 weeks in the first instance and then renewed by the court for periods of up to 28 days at a time to a maximum of one year. The patient does not have to attend court in person when the order is renewed.

This order is also useful for psychiatrists who are uncertain as to whether the individual's mental disorder is going to be amenable to psychiatric treatment, as may occur, for example, in cases of personality disorder.

If, in the end, a Section 37 hospital order is not considered appropriate, then the court can use its discretion to otherwise sentence the individual, including to prison.

Section 41: restriction order

Section 41 (1) states:

> ... where a hospital order is made in respect of an offender by the *Crown Court*, and it appears to the court, having regard to the nature of the offence, the antecedents of the offender and the risk of him committing further offences if set at large, that it is necessary for the *protection of the public from serious harm* so to do, the court may, subject to the provisions of this section, further order the offender shall be subject to special restrictions set out in the section, either without limit of time or during such a period that may be specified in the order; and the order under this section shall be known as a 'Restriction Order'.

It is rare nowadays for the order to be made for a fixed period of time as opposed to 'without limit of time'. This reflects the therapeutic uncertainty of how quickly an individual will progress. One of the two doctors recommending

Section 37 must attend court to give evidence, but it is for the court to decide whether a Section 41 restriction order should be imposed. The main restrictions are that the patient can be discharged absolutely or conditionally, given leave of absence or transferred to another hospital only with the approval of the Home Secretary. A restriction order therefore is an added safeguard, so that the decision to discharge, etc., is not left to the responsible medical officer alone.

If the patient is discharged conditionally, the usual conditions relate to supervision, residence and medical treatment. The main advantage of this order for professionals is that it facilitates the long-term management of mentally abnormal serious offenders by specifying the conditions of their discharge (such as place of residence – e.g. a supervised hostel – and compliance with psychiatric treatment, including medication) upon threat of recall to hospital.

If recalled to hospital, then the individual is subject to a mandatory Mental Health Review Tribunal hearing within the first six months.

Section 37: guardianship order

The grounds for this are as for a Section 37 hospital order. It is used rarely. A proposed guardian must agree to it. If the patient absconds from a place where they are required to live, then he or she may be recaptured and returned there. There are, however, no effective sanctions for a patient refusing to cooperate with psychiatric treatment (such as medication), although attendance to see a psychiatrist can be enforced.

It was hoped in the Butler Report (Home Office and Department of Health and Social Security 1975) that this order might be used increasingly more often, but many social services departments are reluctant to use this order for mentally abnormal offenders, although, again, it can facilitate the management of a mentally abnormal offender in the community.

Section 45A: hospital and limitation directions

This was brought in by the **Crime (Sentences) Act 1997** (see Table 5.2) on 1 October 1997. It is referred to as the 'hybrid order', as it is a prison sentence accompanied by hospital and limitation (equivalent to a restriction order) directions. It is available only to the Crown Court and, currently, only for people suffering from psychopathic disorder.

Written or oral evidence from two doctors is required, and the treatability test applies.

Community rehabilitation orders with a condition of psychiatric treatment

Community rehabilitation orders can be made in any court for any offence other than one with a fixed penalty (such as murder, which carries a mandatory life prison sentence), but they do require conviction. Supervision by a probation officer is for a specified period of between six months and three years.

TABLE 5.2 Mentally disordered offenders and the Crime (Sentences) Act 1997

1 *Mandatory life sentence* for second 'serious offence' (attempted murder, manslaughter, rape, attempted rape) unless exceptional circumstances (which do not include mental disorder alone)

2 *Hospital direction and limitation direction* (equivalent to restriction order) for psychopathic disorder only

   If offender benefits, can serve entire sentence in hospital

3 *Transfers to hospital*

   Court and Home Secretary can specify unit

   Home Secretary's consent required for transfer of restricted patients between hospitals, even if in the same Trust

   Section 47 transfer to mental nursing home now allowed

4 *Interim hospital order*

   Maximum duration extended from 6 months to 1 year

   Can use before a hospital direction

In cases where there is a condition of psychiatric treatment, the court will require evidence from a doctor approved under Section 12 of the Mental Health Act 1983. Conditions may include that the subject receive treatment as an inpatient or in a nursing home and/or as an outpatient at a specified hospital or place from or under the direction of a named doctor.

The court must explain the requirements of the order to the offender and obtain the offender's consent. If the individual subsequently refuses to cooperate with psychiatric treatment, then the doctor can only report this to the supervising probation officer, who may take proceedings on these grounds for breach of the community rehabilitation order. Detention in hospital under the civil provisions of the Mental Health Act 1983 is an alternative disposal, if appropriate, in such circumstances, but it is not a formal court sentence.

AFTER SENTENCING

Transfer direction from prison: Section 47 of the Mental Health Act 1983

This allows the Home Secretary to order the transfer of a sentenced prisoner following conviction if the prisoner is suffering from a mental disorder. The patient is subject to consent to treatment provisions. This order can continue until the earliest date of release, whereupon a notional Section 37 hospital order follows automatically without the need for further completion of legally required medical recommendation reports. Almost inevitably, a restriction direction is also made under Section 49, which has the same effect as a restriction order under Section 41. Such individuals can be returned to prison to complete a sentence before their earliest date of release, e.g. if they recover from their mental illness or they no longer require inpatient treatment. Individuals most frequently transferred from prison on this order are those who develop mental illness during a prison sentence and those in whom the mental illness was missed at the time of sentence.

Transfer of people kept in custody during Her Majesty's Pleasure: Section 46 of the Mental Health Act 1983

This relates to people under the age of 18 years convicted of murder. It also applies to members of the armed forces. It has the same effect as a hospital order with restrictions with no limit of time.

CRIMINAL PROCEEDINGS AND PROPOSED CHANGES OF THE MENTAL HEALTH ACT 1983

The term 'psychopathic disorder' will be subsumed under the general term 'mental disorder'. It is recommended that assessment in hospital for a period up to 12 months ought (but will not have) to be undertaken before a court mental health disposal. It is recommended that there should be a single remand order for both assessment and treatment to be used by Magistrates' and Crown Courts. A compulsory order for care and treatment will apply to whatever setting is deemed appropriate, taking account of public safety, e.g. in the community with a condition of psychiatric treatment. The restriction order is to remain confined for the use of a Crown Court but is not to be linked to the offence. The threat of serious harm to others will remain a key issue. The continuation of compulsory treatment is to be based primarily on risk assessment when mental disorder persists. Access to regular independent Mental Health Tribunals will remain.

PROPOSALS FOR MANAGING DANGEROUS PEOPLE WITH SEVERE PERSONALITY DISORDER (HOME OFFICE 1999)

This recommended that dangerous people with severe personality disorder should be contained in an appropriate setting and not released while they continue to pose a risk to the public. Although a new legal framework to provide paths for the indeterminate detention of dangerous people with severe personality disorder in criminal and civil proceedings and the development of specialist facilities run separately from the prison and health services was originally suggested as an option, it is now planned to develop such services within the framework of current criminal and mental health law, including the new Mental Health Act. Dangerous and severe personality disorder (DSPD) units have already been developed within the health service, e.g. Broadmoor and Rampton special hospitals, and in prisons, e.g. HMP Whitemoor and HMP Frankland.

FORENSIC PSYCHIATRIC ASSESSMENT

See Table 5.3.

TABLE 5.3 Forensic psychiatric assessment

1　Full history and mental state of patient, including fantasies and impulses to offend
2　Objective account of offence, e.g. from arresting police officer or from statements (depositions) in Crown Court cases
3　Objective accounts of past offences, if any, e.g. obtain list of previous convictions
4　Additional information gathering, such as interviews with informants, e.g. relatives, reading a pre-sentence report from a probation officer, if prepared
5　Review of previous psychiatric records, e.g. to ascertain relationship of mental disorder to previous behaviour and response to psychiatric treatment and need for security

PSYCHIATRIC EXPERT EVIDENCE

See Table 5.4.

TABLE 5.4 Psychiatric expert evidence

1　Fitness to plead
2　Mental responsibility, e.g. not guilty by reason of insanity, diminished responsibility
3　Mental disorder, e.g. mental illness, mental impairment, psychopathic disorder
4　Is client treatable?
5　Have arrangements been made for such treatment, e.g. community rehabilitation order with condition of outpatient treatment, or inpatient treatment under Section 37 of Mental Health Act 1983?
6　Is client dangerous, e.g. Section 41 Mental Health Act 1983, placement in a special hospital?
7　Suggestions about non-psychiatric management, e.g. community rehabilitation order, supervised hostel

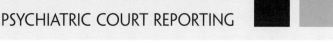

PSYCHIATRIC COURT REPORTING

See Table 5.5.

TABLE 5.5 Court reporting

1   A report may be requested:
    (i)   by a court (Magistrates', Crown or Higher Court), usually through the
          probation service. Written authorization by the court must be given
    (ii) by the defence solicitors, in which case the patient's written permission
          is required before giving a report to solicitors, which remains their
          property to use, or not, in court
2   Information required for a report includes:
    (i)   information about the charge
    (ii) pre-sentence report from a probation officer
    (iii) list of previous convictions
    (iv) previous medical hospital notes
    (v)   previous reports (social and medical)
    (vi) depositions where available, e.g. Crown Court but not Magistrates'
          Court cases
3   The history will be taken from the patient and, if possible, a relative or
    friend
4   The client should be fully examined physically
5   The questions that the court or solicitor will be particularly interested in
    are:
    (i)   does the patient have a mental disorder?
    (ii) is the disorder susceptible to or requiring specific treatment?
    (iii) can arrangements be made for such treatment (hospital, outpatient,
          etc.)?
    (iv) is the patient dangerous?
    (v)   have you any suggestions as to the patient's management, apart from
          the psychiatric aspects?
6   After interview and examination of other reports, etc., one can valuably
    discuss the case again with the probation officer or others, e.g. other
    psychiatrists, involved in the case
    (i)   discuss in particular your findings and compare them with other
          professionals' observations, which may reveal gross discrepancies
    (ii) discussion may reveal unexpected channels for disposal or unforeseen
          difficulties
7   The general principles of the written report are:
    (i)   it should be in clear English, and technical terms should be avoided if
          possible. If such terms are used, then an explanation of them should
          be given, e.g. paranoid (persecutory) delusions (false beliefs), auditory
          and visual hallucinations (voices and visions)
    (ii) use the report to help the court reach the most appropriate disposal
          for the patient
    (iii) the report is a recommendation to the court. The court may have other
          psychiatric opinions that oppose yours and may itself be unconvinced

TABLE 5.5 cont'd. Court reporting

by your opinion. Thus, the onus is on you to provide the evidence in the report for your opinion

(iv) the onus is also on the reporting doctor to make all the necessary medical arrangements for the disposal and management of the patient

(v) be accurate, complete and brief. The court is extremely busy and will resent a turgid, overwritten report. For Magistrates' Courts, which may deal with dozens of cases a day, about two pages may suffice and, even then, only the opinion may be read

8   People use different forms for their report, but the following is suggested. Paragraph numbers and headings can be used for clarity

Paragraph 1: introduction

Inform the court of when and where the patient was seen, and at whose request, what information was available, who the informants were, and (sometimes) what information was not available. State the current offence(s) for which the patient is charged, the date of the offence(s), and the plea, if known (i.e. guilty or not guilty).

Paragraph 2: past medical history

Inform the court of this and of the result of medical examination, e.g. 'Physical examination revealed no abnormality'.

Paragraph 3: family history

Report the important, relevant points, including family history (or not) of psychiatric disorder and criminality.

Paragraph 4: personal history

Report the important points of his physical development, e.g. birth and milestones, early development, e.g. bedwetting (enuresis), schooling, e.g. truancy, and occupational history, which could include difficulties at work, e.g. sackings, or in sustaining employment, or with colleagues or supervisors at work.

Paragraph 5: sexual history

Be reasonably discreet: the report may be read in open court.

Paragraph 6: previous personality

Report details of personality in terms of social interaction, emotions and habits, e.g. drinking, gambling and drugs.

Paragraph 7: past forensic history

Technically, past convictions should not be admissible before conviction, but they are admissible when the report is to assist in sentencing. In practice, sometimes only one psychiatric report is prepared for both trial and sentencing.

Paragraph 8: past psychiatric history

Report dates, diagnosis, relevant details and relationship of mental disorder and treatment to offending.

TABLE 5.5 cont'd. Court reporting

Paragraph 9: circumstances surrounding index offence(s)

Report circumstances leading to current offence(s) and defendant's state of mind at the time of the offence, sticking to the phenomena reported, e.g. 'for the time of the offence, he gives a history of tearfulness, loss of hope, poor sleeping …'; ' … these are symptoms of a depressive mental illness …'

Paragraph 10: interview

Report the result of the interview, e.g. 'He showed/did not show evidence of mental illness'. Then give a brief outline of the evidence, e.g. 'He muttered to himself and looked around the room as though hearing voices (auditory hallucinations) …', or list the symptoms and say, for example, 'these are symptoms of the severe mental illness of schizophrenia'.

Information in Paragraphs 1–10 should be factual, verifiable and, ideally, agreed by all, even if others' opinions differ from your own.

Paragraph 11: opinion

The final paragraph should express your opinion. The court will be interested particularly in your opinion as to:

(a) Is he fit to plead and stand his trial
(b) Is he suffering from a mental illness, a form of mental impairment or psychopathic disorder
(c) If so, can arrangements be made for his treatment (Fix this up if you can). Make suggestions to the court about which disposal would be appropriate, e.g., Section 37 hospital order with or without a Section 41 restriction order, outpatient psychiatric treatment as a condition of a Community Rehabilitation Order.

For example:

'This man is fit to plead and stand trial.

In my opinion he suffers from the severe mental illness of schizophrenia, characterized by delusions (false beliefs) of passivity (being externally controlled) and auditory hallucinations (voices) talking about him in a derogatory way in the third person.

I consider he would benefit from treatment in a psychiatric hospital. I have made arrangements for a bed to be reserved for him at X hospital under Section 37 of the Mental Health Act 1983 if the court considers that this would be appropriate.

I recommend, if the court so agrees, that he additionally be made subject to restrictions under Section 41 of the Mental Health Act 1983 to protect the public from serious harm and to facilitate his long-term psychiatric management, including by specifying the conditions of his discharge from hospital e.g., of residence, and compliance with outpatient treatment, and by providing the ability to recall him to hospital should his mental state or behaviour deteriorate or he otherwise gives rise to concern.'

OR, as an alternative:

'In my opinion this man does not suffer from mental illness, mental impairment nor psychopathic disorder and is not detainable in hospital under the Mental

TABLE 5.5 cont'd. Court reporting

Health Act 1983. He has an immature personality and requires considerable
support and would benefit from group psychotherapy as an out-patient. If the
court is prepared to consider an alternative to a custodial sentence in this case,
I would recommend that, subject to the probation service's agreement, he be
made subject to the direction of a Community Rehabilitation Order with a
condition that he attend an outpatient group under my direction at X Mental
Health Unit.'

Express any doubts you may have as to the likelihood of benefit from or risks
associated with treatment in this man's case.

If you have no psychiatric recommendation, say so, e.g., 'I have no psychiatric
recommendation to make in this case.'

Finally, if essential information is lacking or if time is not sufficient to make the
necessary arrangements for a hospital bed, then do not hesitate to state your
findings to date, state what you would like to do, and ask for a further period of
remand.

REFERENCES

Dell, S (1984). *Murder into Manslaughter: The Diminished Responsibility Defence in Practice (Maudsley Monographs)*. Oxford: Oxford University Press.

Home Office and Department of Health and Social Security (1975). *Report of the Committee on Mentally Abnormal Offenders (Butler Report)*. London: HMSO.

Consent to treatment

ETHICAL PRINCIPLES AND CONSENT

Introduction

Ethical principles underlie the practice of medicine and provide a guide for difficult and painful decisions about human behaviour. This is particularly relevant in psychiatry, as decisions about restricting individual freedom through mental health legislation routinely occur in this specialty. Also, decisions about administering medication to patients who are not thought to be competent to decide on their treatment have to be taken regularly.

Many factors in today's society create conflicting demands on physicians. These include advances in scientific research, civil rights and consumer movements, increased public education, effects of the law on medicine, pressure of economy, and moral, religions and ethnic dilemmas. These require a clear understanding of the guiding ethical principles as well as a knowledge of the relevant medical practice.

Autonomy

Informed consent is the cornerstone of the ethical theory of autonomy, which is based on the writings of Immanuel Kant. This theory describes the relationship between a physician and a normal adult patient as a relationship between two responsible people rather than between a parent and a child. This is the theory that the law tends to recognize, and its assumption of the adult's competence, the right to informed consent in treatment and research, the right to refuse treatment, and limitations on a psychiatrist's ability to hospitalize involuntarily can be seen as recognition of an adult's fundamental right to self-determination in medical decision-making. This is, however, sometimes in direct opposition to society's expectations concerning people with mental health problems and their perceived dangerousness.

Adult patients are presumed to have the right and capacity to consent or refuse consent to treatment. However, the effects of illness and particularly mental disorder may confuse the issue.

Definition of consent

Consent is the voluntary permission of the patient to a particular treatment or procedure. This can be withdrawn at any time and is based on information given to the patient for the purpose of the treatment. What it entails, likely effects and side-effects, alternatives to that treatment, and consequences of refusal should be explained, e.g. amputation of a gangrenous limb and consequences of non-amputation.

Medical treatment

In the context of mental health legislation, medical treatment refers to the broad range of activities aimed at alleviating or preventing a deterioration of a patient's mental disorder. It includes:

- nursing care
- other forms of care
- habilitation
- rehabilitation
- electroconvulsive therapy (ECT)
- administration of drugs
- psychotherapy.

Treatment plans are essential for informal and detained patients alike. Consultant psychiatrists should coordinate the formulation of the treatment plan in consultation with their other professional colleagues and *record* it.

Before an individual can be given medical treatment, his or her valid consent is required, except in cases in which the law provides authority to treat the patient without consent.

Types of consent

There are two main types of consent:

- implied consent
- express consent.

Implied consent

Implied consent occurs in the normal course of contact between a clinical professional and a patient. For example, a patient actively indicates consent by holding out their arm for a blood test or rolling up their sleeve to allow their blood pressure to be taken. This form of consent is used where risk is low and there is minimal invasiveness.

Express consent

Express consent is either verbal or written consent and should be obtained for procedures where there is a risk and a degree of invasiveness, such as in an operation for hernia.

Treatment without consent

In general, in medicine and psychiatry treatment may be given to a patient only with his or her valid consent. Note that there are two components to this: the patient must give his or her consent, and the consent must be valid. Failure to fulfil either part is generally illegal (unless it is covered by common law or by, for

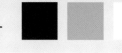

example, the Mental Health Act – see below) and may constitute battery or negligence, respectively.

Battery

Battery is a trespass against the person and occurs if treatment is given to a patient without his or her consent (where not otherwise authorized, e.g. by the Mental Health Act).

Negligence

It is not sufficient to obtain the consent of a patient to a treatment in the absence of reasonable explanation (*Chatterton* v. *Gerson and another* (1980)); such an action may be construed as being negligent.

Reasons why treatment may need to be given without consent

The position is that treatment can be given without consent when the patient is incapable of giving consent because he or she:

- is a child: in this case, the parent or guardian consents (unless the child is aged 16 years or over or is Gillick-competent);
- is unconscious and is in urgent need of treatment to preserve life, health or wellbeing (unless there is a previous refusal of such treatment);
- is suffering from a mental disorder and is incapable;
- is otherwise incapable and is in need of medical care in circumstances in which the patient has not declared unwillingness to be treated before he or she became incapable.

In all of these cases, the treatment, to be lawful, must be in the patient's best interests (see below). Note that the common law applies to all patients, informal or detained, except in those situations in which the Mental Health Act specifically overrides it.

Best interests

Decisions taken on behalf of a person lacking capacity require careful assessment of that person as an individual. Although at the time of writing there is no statutory guidance on the meaning of 'best interests', there is a proposed statutory checklist in the Draft Mental Incapacity Bill. Clause 4 of the draft Bill seeks to establish the common-law principle that any act done for, or any decision made on behalf of, a person who lacks capacity must be in the person's 'best interests'. This principle has become well-established and developed by the courts in cases relating to incapacitated adults. Under the draft Bill, capacity to do the act or make the decision in question must first be assessed, and Clause 4 comes into play only once it has been established that the person lacks capacity. It then sets out a number of basic common factors to which 'regard must be had' in all situations when determining what is in an incapacitated person's best interests. Clause 4, on 'best interests', reads as follows:

(1) Where under this Act any act is done for, or any decision is made on behalf of, a person who lacks capacity, the act must be done or the decision made in the person's best interests.

(2) In deciding for the purposes of this Act what is in a person's best interests, regard must be had to

(a) whether he is likely to have capacity in relation to the matter in question in the future;

(b) the need to permit and encourage him to participate, or to improve his ability to participate, as fully as possible in any act done for and any decision affecting him;

(c) so far as ascertainable
(i)   his past and present wishes and feelings, and
(ii) the factors which he would consider if he were able to do so;

(d) if it is practicable and appropriate to consult them, the views of
(i)   any person named by him as someone to be consulted on the matter in question or on matters of that kind,
(ii) any person engaged in caring for him or interested in his welfare,
(iii) any donee of a lasting power of attorney granted by him, and
(iv) any deputy appointed for him by the court,

as to his past and present wishes and feelings and the factors he would consider if he were able to do so;

(e) whether the purpose for which any act or decision is needed can be as effectively achieved in a way less restrictive of his freedom of action.

(3) The duty in subsection (1) also applies in relation to the exercise of any powers which under this Act are exercisable
(a) under a lasting power of attorney, or
(b) in circumstances where it is reasonably believed that a person lacks capacity.

(4) In the case of an act done, or a decision made, by a person other than the court, there is sufficient compliance with subsection (1) if the person reasonably believes that what he does or decides is in the best interests of the person concerned.

Situations requiring consent

The following situations require consent:

- medical and nursing procedures;
- mental health treatment;
- photography, videoing, filming, etc.;
- the presence of students for teaching or work experience;
- human immunodeficiency virus (HIV) testing;
- genetic testing.

ABILITY TO CONSENT

In order to be able to consent, a patient must be able to:

- communicate a choice;
- understand and retain relevant information about the proposed medical treatment and treatment alternatives;

- appreciate his or her clinical situation, and believe it;
- manipulate information rationally, i.e. weigh it up and make a choice.

Mood (affective) disorders and decision-making

A patient who feels worthless may refuse treatment out of a desire to cease to be a burden. A hopeless patient may believe that a bad outcome, although statistically unlikely, is certain to occur in his or her case.

Cognitive impairment and decision-making

Some people suffering from dementia may still be able to make valid decisions. However, many will not be able to understand the situation, and although they may be able to appreciate that something is wrong, this realization does not last and they are often unable to manipulate the information.

Psychiatric disorders in general

Patients may not be capable of consenting; this is a matter for exercising clinical judgement guided by current professional practice and subject to legal requirements when it comes to making decisions for them.

The presence of a mental disorder such as schizophrenia does not necessarily mean that the person is incapable of giving valid consent, but the presence of delusions may mean that the person cannot satisfy the complete criteria for informed consent.

CAPACITY TO CONSENT

Capacity to consent may be variable, and patients are more likely to be able to give valid consent if the information is pitched at an appropriate level, e.g. written and verbal information should be given in broad terms and simple language. In the case of an illiterate person, a tape-recording of the verbal discussion might be helpful.

Capacity to consent for a particular individual should be assessed at a specific time for a particular treatment and may vary according to mental state.

The information given should include the relevant current medical knowledge and practice. In every case, enough information should be given to ensure that the patient understands in broad terms the nature, likely effects and risks of the treatment, including the likelihood of success and alternatives to it. A two-way discussion is a useful way of understanding that the patient comprehends the entire treatment fully.

There may be a good reason for withholding information when it is in the patient's best interests, but the person withholding the facts must be able to be justify why all information was not disclosed and the doctor must make it clear that he or she is not answering a patient's questions in their entirety. The doctor must be truthful.

The patient should be informed that consent can be withdrawn at any time and that fresh consent is required before further treatment is instigated.

CAPACITY TO MAKE A DECISION

It is presumed in common law that an adult has full legal capacity unless it is shown that he or she does not. Should anybody challenge this, the onus is on them to prove that, on the balance of probabilities, the patient is incapable.

The principles of capacity are that the person must be able to understand what the treatment is, that somebody has said that he or she needs it, and why it is being proposed. The patient must understand in broad terms the nature of the treatment, e.g. where scars will occur and the likelihood of pain after an operation. In particular, the following criteria should be fulfilled:

- The patient must understand the principal benefits and risks of the treatment, e.g. in respect of a colostomy instead of a simple bowel operation.
- The patient must understand the consequences of not receiving the proposed treatment.

An assessment of capability has to be made concerning a particular treatment plan. Capacity in an individual with a mental disorder is variable over time. All assessments of capacity should be recorded fully in the patient's medical notes.

INCAPACITY AND MEDICAL TREATMENT

Patients who are incapable of making a decision are usually unable to understand information. Giving medical treatment to people incapable of consenting to the treatment is a big step and causes concern. However, people who are incapable may still require treatment, and it is not reasonable that this be denied to them; moreover, consideration needs to be given to the duty to treat.

The House of Lords' decision in *Re F* (1989) 2 WLR 1025 (1989) 2 All ER 545 helped to clarify the common-law situation with regard to general medical and surgical treatment of people who lack capacity to give consent. This decision said that a doctor may lawfully operate on or give treatment to a person who lacks the capacity to give consent provided that it is in the best interests of the patient, i.e. to save life, to prevent deterioration, or to ensure an improvement in his or her physical or mental health. If necessary, the doctors should seek the advice of a court before proceeding with procedures such as sterilization.

REFUSAL TO CONSENT

Duty to patient

The right to refuse treatment is not a right to be killed. A person is completely at liberty to decline to undergo treatment, even if the result of his or her doing so will be that he or she will die.

The doctor owes a duty to the patient. The competent patient, by giving consent to treatment, seeks the help of the doctor. If the doctor has undertaken to treat by accepting the person as a patient, then the doctor has a duty to treat. A patient's consent cannot justify that which the law forbids, e.g. the direct taking of life or acting contrary to clinical judgement.

Persistent vegetative state

There is a need for a decision-making procedure for patients who are unconscious or quite unable to express any decision although they may not be suffering from any condition that could be construed as a mental illness (*Airedale NHS Trust* v. *Bland* (1993) AC 789).

Verbal but not written consent

Verbal consent is unusual, but occasionally it can be given. When given, a record should be entered into the patient's case file. A signed contract is the only evidence of agreement between a professional and a patient.

Lack of consent to full treatment

Patients may not consent in full to a treatment or procedure, e.g. the patient may agree to a lump being removed from a breast but not a full mastectomy. It is important that this is adhered to.

INCAPACITY OR INABILITY TO MAKE A DECISION

The assessor must consider the patient's ability to understand information and to use this information in exercising choice. The first guidance on the question of capacity and medical treatment was *Re C (adult refusal of treatment)*. The judge found it useful to look at capacity as follows:

- comprehending and retaining information;
- believing it;
- weighing it up to make a choice.

It has been suggested that a person should be found to lack capacity if he or she is not able to comprehend an explanation of the problem in broad terms and simple language. People should not be found to lack capacity necessarily if the decision that they arrive at would not have been made by someone of ordinary prudence.

PROCESS OF OBTAINING CONSENT

The process of obtaining informed consent should include enough time and information to enable the person to make an informed choice about his or her proposed treatment. It is important that consent for an operation gives the patient sufficient time to weigh up the information. Similarly, if a period of time elapses between consent and treatment and the patient's condition alters, consent should be taken again. Consent should be obtained by a person familiar with all aspects of the treatment, including the risks and alternatives. This is usually a senior doctor.

The process requires good communication skills, trust, respect and rapport between the patient and the professional. Written material and diagrams, if necessary, can be helpful. Considerable care needs to be taken to ensure that the patient understands the information. The process may need to be repeated more than once: the consent the person is giving may be something he or she is worried about, as they may have been subjected to false information, such as from old wives' tales or from other patients who have had the treatment.

Attention should also be paid to communicating fully with people with hearing and sight difficulties. Interpreters should be arranged for patients whose first language is not English. It is not a good idea to involve a relative in translating, as this can interfere with the patient's autonomy. A record should be made in the patient's file of the discussion, and any particular preferences or concerns the patient may have must be noted carefully.

The professional should confirm again that the patient understands the material.

GUIDELINES TO PATIENTS FROM THE DEPARTMENT OF HEALTH

The Department of Health has issued the following information to patients relating to consent:

ABOUT THE CONSENT FORM

Before a doctor or other health professional examines or treats you, they need your consent. Sometimes you can simply tell them whether you agree with their suggestions. However, sometimes a written record of your decision is helpful – for example if your treatment involves sedation or general anaesthesia. You'll then be asked to sign a consent form. If you later change your mind, you're entitled to withdraw consent – even after signing.

WHAT SHOULD I KNOW BEFORE DECIDING?

Health professionals must ensure you know enough to enable you to decide about treatment. They'll write information on the consent form and offer

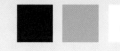
you a copy to keep as well as discussing the choices of treatment with you. Although they may well recommend a particular option, you're free to choose another. People's attitudes vary on things like the amount of risk or pain they're prepared to accept. That goes for the amount of information, too. If you'd rather not know about certain aspects, discuss your worries with whoever is treating you.

SHOULD I ASK QUESTIONS?

Always ask anything you want. As a reminder, you can write your questions in the space over the page. The person you ask should do his or her best to answer, but if they don't know they should find someone else who is able to discuss your concerns. To support you and prompt questions, you might like to bring a friend or relative. Ask if you'd like someone independent to speak up for you.

IS THERE ANYTHING I SHOULD TELL PEOPLE?

If there's any procedure you don't want to happen, you should tell the people treating you. It's also important for them to know about any illnesses or allergies which you may have or have suffered from in the past.

CAN I FIND OUT MORE ABOUT GIVING CONSENT?

The Department of Health leaflet *Consent – what you have a right to expect* is a detailed guide on consent in versions for adults, children, parents, carers/relatives and people with learning disabilities. Ask for one from your clinic or hospital, order one from the NHS Responseline (08701 555 455) or read it on the web site www.doh.gov.uk/consent.

WHO IS TREATING ME?

Amongst the health professionals treating you may be a 'doctor in training' – medically qualified, but now doing more specialist training. They range from recently qualified doctors to doctors almost ready to be consultants. They will only carry out procedures for which they have been appropriately trained. Someone senior will supervise – either in person accompanying a less experienced doctor in training or available to advise someone more experienced.

WHAT ABOUT ANAESTHESIA?

If your treatment involves general or regional anaesthesia (where more than a small part of your body is being anaesthetised), you'll be given general information about it in advance. You'll also have an opportunity to talk with the anaesthetist when he or she assesses your state of health shortly before treatment. Hospitals sometimes have pre-assessment clinics which provide patients with the chance to discuss things a few weeks earlier.

WILL SAMPLES BE TAKEN?

Some kinds of operation involve removing a part of the body (such as a gall bladder or a tooth). You would always be told about this in advance. Other operations may mean taking samples as part of your care. These samples may be of blood or small sections of tissue, for example of an unexplained lump. Such samples may be further checked by other health professionals to ensure the best possible standards. Again, you should be told in advance if samples are likely to be taken.

Sometimes samples taken during operations may also be used for teaching, research or public health monitoring in the future interests of all NHS patients. The NHS Trust treating you will have a local system for checking whether you're willing for this to happen.

PHOTOGRAPHS AND VIDEOS

As part of your treatment some kind of photographic record may be made – for example X-rays, clinical photographs or sometimes a video. You will always be told if this is going to happen. The photograph or recording will be kept with your notes and will be held in confidence as part of your medical record. This means that it will normally be seen only by those involved in providing you with care or those who need to check the quality of care you have received. The use of photographs and recordings is also extremely important for other NHS work, such as teaching or medical research. However, we will not use yours in a way that might allow you to be identified or recognised without your express permission.

WHAT IF THINGS DON'T GO AS EXPECTED?

Amongst the 25,000 operations taking place every day, sometimes things don't go as they should. Although the doctor involved should inform you and your family, often the patient is the first to notice something amiss. If you're worried – for example about the after-effects of an operation continuing much longer than you were told to expect – tell a health professional right away. Speak to your GP, or contact your clinic – the phone number should be on your appointment card, letter or consent form copy.

WHAT ARE THE KEY THINGS TO REMEMBER?

It's your decision! It's up to you to choose whether or not to consent to what's being proposed. Ask as many questions as you like, and remember to

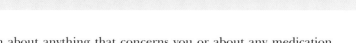

tell the team about anything that concerns you or about any medication, allergies or past history which might affect your general health.

QUESTIONS TO ASK HEALTH PROFESSIONALS

As well as giving you information health professionals must listen and do their best to answer your questions. Before your next appointment, you can write some down in the space below. Questions may be about the treatment itself, for example:

- What are the main treatment options?
- What are the benefits of each of the options?
- What are the risks, if any, of each option?
- What are the success rates for different options – nationally, for this unit or for you (the surgeon)?
- Why do you think an operation (if suggested) is necessary?
- What are the risks if I decide to do nothing for the time being?
- How can I expect to feel after the procedure?
- When am I likely to be able to get back to work?

Questions may also be about how the treatment might affect your future state of health or style of life, for example:

- Will I need long-term care?
- Will my mobility be affected?
- Will I still be able to drive?
- Will it affect the kind of work I do?
- Will it affect my personal/sexual relationships?
- Will I be able to take part in my favourite sport/exercises?
- Will I be able to follow my usual diet?

Health care professionals should welcome your views and discuss any issues so they can work in partnership with you for the best outcome.

THE MENTAL HEALTH ACT 1983 AND CONSENT

Part IV of the Mental Health Act 1983

Part IV of the Mental Health Act 1983 is concerned with the issue of consent to treatment and applies to any patient liable to be detained under this Act, *except*:

- a patient detained (for up to 72 hours) in an emergency under Section 4;
- an informal patient detained (for up to 72 hours) under Section 5(2) to prevent him or her from leaving the hospital;
- an informal patient detained (for up to 6 hours) under Section 5(4) to prevent him or her from leaving hospital;

- an accused person remanded to hospital by a court for a report on his or her mental condition, under Section 35;
- a patient believed to be suffering from mental disorder and who is detained (for up to 72 hours) in a place of safety under Section 135;
- a person found in a public place and who appears to be suffering from mental disorder who is removed by the police and detained (for up to 72 hours) in a place of safety under Section 136;
- a convicted patient detained (for up to 28 days) in a place of safety and awaiting transfer to hospital under Section 37;
- a patient who has been conditionally discharged under section 42, 73 or 74 and who has not been recalled to hospital.

Treatment requiring consent and a second opinion (Section 57)

The treatments that come under the umbrella of Section 57 of the Mental Health Act 1983 are psycho-surgery and implantation of sex hormones. These cannot be carried out without the capable patient's consent and a second opinion.

Treatment requiring consent or second opinion (Section 58)

This section covers physical treatments of mental disorder, including medication (after the first three months) and ECT.

Patients can be treated for three months on medication for their mental disorder without their consent. This does not apply to medical treatment for physical illness, to which common law applies.

In the case of ECT, this treatment entails taking blood samples. Similarly, in the situation where lithium treatment is used, thyroid function and creatinine clearance monitoring and serum lithium levels in guidance with the *British National Formulary* (BNF) can be carried out. With regard to clozapine administration, this will also include regular venepuncture.

Urgent treatment (Section 62)

In respect of urgent treatment covered by Section 57 or Section 58, under Section 62 of the Mental Health Act 1983 it is the case that the safeguards set out in sections 57 and 58 do not apply to any of the following cases:

- the treatment is immediately necessary to save the patient's life;
- the treatment, not being irreversible, is immediately necessary to prevent a serious deterioration of the patient's condition;
- the treatment, not being irreversible or hazardous, is immediately necessary to alleviate serious suffering by the patient;
- the treatment, not being irreversible or hazardous, is immediately necessary and represents the minimum interference necessary to prevent the patient from behaving violently or being a danger to him- or herself or to others.

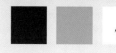

Irreversible treatment

For the purposes of Section 62, a treatment is irreversible if it has unfavourable irreversible physical or psychological consequences (Section 62, Subsection 3).

Hazardous treatment

For the purposes of Section 62, a treatment is hazardous if it entails significant physical hazard (Section 62, Subsection 3).

7

Mental health, medication and the law

INTRODUCTION

The reason for administration of medication to a patient suffering from a mental disorder is similar to that for the administration of medication for any other disorder. This is to alleviate or control the suffering that the person is experiencing and to cure the underlying condition that is causing the patient to suffer. The patient should have the capacity to consent to taking the medication. He or she should have been provided with information in sufficient detail to enable him or her to make a decision based on an adequate knowledge of the nature, purpose, likely effects and risks of the medication, including the likelihood of its success and any alternatives to it. The patient is free to refuse the medication if he or she wishes.

There is, however, a difference in the case of a patient detained under the Mental Health Act 1983, when they may not, because of their symptoms, accept the need for medication and therefore not consent to receive it. Many detained patients are, nevertheless, capable of consenting to take medication, but some are incapable of doing so.

MENTAL HEALTH ACT 1983

The administration of medication to detained patients is subject to the provisions of Part IV of the Act, and this is discussed in Chapter 6. Section 63 provides that a patient to whom Part IV of the Act applies may, without his or her consent and without any other independent permission, be given medication for their mental disorder during the first three months of their treatment, provided that it is given by or under the direction of the responsible medical officer (RMO).

Section 58 of the Mental Health Act 1983 refers to treatment for a mental disorder, which requires either the compulsorily detained person's consent or a second-opinion appointed doctor (SOAD) from the Mental Health Commission. This includes electroconvulsive therapy (ECT) given at any time and the administration of medicine once three months have elapsed since medication was first given.

A statutory certificate must be completed. In the case of a patient who is able to understand the nature, purpose and likely effects of a treatment and has consented to it, a Form 38 must be completed. This states which psychotropic medications are to be given and whether the doses conform to the *British National Formulary* (BNF) guideline doses.

In the event that the patient does not understand the nature, purpose or likely effects of the treatment, or does not consent to it, the SOAD has to complete a Form 39. This occurs after discussing the care plan with the RMO and another non-nursing professional involved in the patient's care. The SOAD should then agree that the treatment that the RMO is proposing is not unreasonable. There has been a challenge to the working of SOADs under the Human Rights Act 1998, in which the SOAD procedure was challenged under Article 8 of the Convention. This states 'individuals have a right to integrity of person and self determination under the Common Law', but these rights are infringed by medical treatment in the absence of consent and require a hearing by a fair and impartial court according to Article 6(1). The guidelines to SOADs are such that they should not substitute their own opinion for that of the RMO but should decide if the latter's decision is 'reasonable in the light of the general consensus of appropriate treatment for such a condition'. The SOAD therefore does not become a judicial or quasi-judicial body deciding upon the lawfulness of a treatment on its merits. The case was discontinued and was not determined fully in court.

In the case of *R (Wilkinson)* v. *Responsible Medical Officer, Broadmoor Hospital and others* (2001), in which a decision to administer medical treatment to a psychiatric patient without his consent under Section 58(3)(b) of the Mental Health Act 1983 was challenged by way of judicial review, the court was entitled to reach its own view as to the merits of the medical decision and whether this decision infringed the patient's human rights. The patient had been detained compulsorily following conviction for the rape of a girl in 1967. In 1999, the patient's RMO at Broadmoor Hospital decided that the patient should receive treatment with antipsychotic medication, in spite of his refusal to consent, pursuant to sections 58(3)(b)(4) and 63 of the Mental Health Act 1983. The patient argued that this decision infringed his rights under articles 2, 3 and 8 of the Convention for the Protection of Human Rights and Fundamental Freedoms and that Article 6 imposed a duty on the court to investigate the facts of the case (and not just the issue of whether the decision was reasonable). The court stated that following the Human Rights Act 1998 coming into force, and given that the prospective Convention breaches either were fundamental or raised issues of necessity or proportionality, there was a clear need for the court to investigate the medical issues. The court would have to reach its own view on whether the patient was capable of consenting to treatment and whether such treatment would endanger his life in breach of Article 2, be degrading in breach of Article 3, or an invasion of his privacy under Article 8, which could not be justified as necessary or proportionate. The court also stated that Article 6 did not entitle every patient to challenge a treatment plan before being subjected to it any more than it entitled a criminal to pre-empt arrest by challenging the constable's right to arrest him. A medically justifiable decision to administer forcible treatment without forewarning the patient did not of itself involve any violation of Article 6.

Section 62 is used if urgent treatment for mental disorder is needed for a compulsorily detained patient. As explained in Chapter 6, this will happen if the treatment in question:

- is immediately necessary to save the patient's life;
- not being irreversible, is immediately necessary to prevent a serious deterioration in the patient's condition;
- not being irreversible or hazardous, is immediately necessary to alleviate serious suffering by the patient;
- not being irreversible or hazardous, is immediately necessary to prevent the patient from behaving violently or from being a danger to him- or herself or others.

Under Section 62(3), for the purposes of Section 62 treatment is considered irreversible if it has unfavourable irreversible physical or psychological consequences, and considered hazardous if it entails significant physical hazard. For example, a treatment such as ECT may be hazardous for an aged person or a person who has an anaesthetic risk.

MISUSE OF DRUGS REGULATIONS 2001

The **Misuse of Drugs Act 1971** led to the **Misuse of Drugs Regulations 1985**. These govern how controlled drugs are supplied and stored. There were nine amendments to these regulations, which have now been consolidated into the **Misuse of Drugs Regulations 2001**; the earlier legislation has been revoked. The main change in the 2001 regulations is that unauthorized possession of benzodiazepines, including possession without a prescription, is now an offence.

Schedule 1

Schedule 1 controlled drugs include the hallucinogenic drugs ecstasy, LSD and cannabis. A Home Office licence is required for legal possession of these drugs. Currently, the only exemption occurs when a professional removes the drug from a person for the purpose of destruction or handing to the police, and this should be witnessed by another professional and documented. There are currently suggestions from some quarters that the controls on cannabis and ecstasy may be relaxed by moving to Schedule 2.

Some cannabis extracts are being used in clinical trials for pain in multiple sclerosis and in terminal illnesses, but currently the relevant centres have Home Office licences to cover this work.

Schedule 2

Schedule 2 drugs include the opiates, major stimulants and secobarbital. All except secobarbital need specified secure storage. The method of destruction and the essential witnesses of the process are laid out in the regulations.

Schedule 3

Schedule 3 drugs include most of the barbiturates (except secobarbital, which is in Schedule 2), buprenorphine, flunitrazepam, temazepam and others. Words

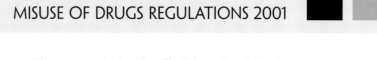

and figures are required when writing a prescription for all of them (see below), except for temazepam and phenobarbital. There are also safe-storage requirements for buprenorphine and the benzodiazepines, but registers are not required legally; some hospitals have opted to have them for all Schedule 3 drugs to avoid confusion.

Schedule 4

Schedule 4 drugs include the remaining benzodiazepines and various hormonal products that are prone to abuse. These may be prescribed and stored in the same way as ordinary prescription-only drugs.

Schedule 5

Schedule 5 drugs include preparations such as kaolin and morphine mixture and codeine tablets. Their abuse potential is lessened by their formulation, and they are treated as ordinary medications.

Prescription of controlled drugs

An example of a prescription for controlled drugs can be found at the front of the BNF, describing how the prescription is to be written in the prescriber's own handwriting with the quantity in both words and figures. The prescription must be signed and dated by the prescriber and must specify the prescriber's address. The prescription should be in ink or otherwise in a form that is indelible.

Words and figures are not required for hospital inpatient drug charts if the drug involved is held as stock on that ward. A ward register is not required by these guidelines but is required by Department of Health guidelines.

Drug-administration errors

There are a number of ways in which harm may occur to a patient in the course of drug administration:

■ *Errors on the prescription sheet:*
  – wrong drug
  – wrong dose
  – drug prescribed leads to side-effects or drug interactions
  – patient is allergic to drug
  – writing is illegible.

■ *Wrong drug dispensed:*
  – wrong patient (similar name)
  – wrong dose
  – failure to note dangerous drug interaction
  – difficulty due to illegible writing.

■ *Error in administration:*

– wrong time
– wrong patient, not checked with prescription card
– wrong amount of drug given
– wrong drug
– wrong route of administration
– drug not given.

It is estimated that there are 850 000 incidents of drug administration errors per annum (National Patient Safety Agency) in hospitals in the UK. A pilot study by the National Patient Safety Agency in 18 NHS Trust hospitals over a nine-month period identified 2514 errors, of which 12 (0.5%) were classified as major or catastrophic (Department of Health 2004). These occur for a variety of reasons. Errors of prescribing can occur if the wrong drug is written down, or if the correct drug but in the wrong dose is written down, e.g. heparin 25 000 units when 2500 units were intended. Another source of prescribing error is the addition of another drug to a patient's medications and the former interacting dangerously with one of the latter, e.g. prescribing a tricyclic antidepressant when a patient is already taking a monoamine oxidase inhibitor (MAOI).

There is scope for a prescription to be misinterpreted if it is not written carefully. The heparin error described above has also occurred when the prescriber wrote '2500 u' and the nurse administering it misread the 'u' as a zero. The BNF recommends that the word 'units' should always be written in full for this reason. Also, doses smaller than 1 mg should be written in micrograms, e.g. digoxin 62.5 micrograms, not 0.0625 mg. There have been numerous incidents of doctors writing 0.625 mg by mistake and of nurses miscalculating the conversion.

Abbreviations can also be misinterpreted, e.g. ISDN 10 mg (isosorbide denigrate) has been dispensed as Istin 10 mg. (Istin® is the commercial name in the UK for Pfizer's preparation of the calcium-channel blocker amlodipine). Similarly, the abbreviation AZT (the antiviral drug azidothymidine or zidovudine) has been misinterpreted as azathioprine (an antiproliferative immuno-suppressant), with fatal consequences.

Dispensing errors can occur if the pharmacist selects the wrong drug from the shelf because of similar names or similar packaging. Another error is the possibility that the correct drug can be supplied labelled with the wrong dose. Also, the correct drug and dose but the wrong patient's name can be on the label.

Errors in administration can occur when a drug is given to the wrong patient. The wrong amount can also be given owing to a miscalculation of the volume of the liquid, because the amount of medication per millilitre is not standardized and has to be worked out for each substance.

Intravenous administration and intrathecal administration have been confused in the case of vincristine, with tragic results. The vinca alkaloids vincristine, vinblastine, vindesine and vinorelbine are chemotherapeutic agents that are for intravenous administration only; intrathecal administration leads to severe neurotoxicity, which usually is fatal.

NATIONAL PATIENT SAFETY AGENCY

This is an independent National Health Service (NHS) body created to coordinate the efforts of all those involved in healthcare and, more importantly, to learn from adverse incidents occurring in the NHS. There are bound to be mistakes when many people receive numerous different medications without any standards or systems in place. This organization aims to promote an open and fair culture in hospitals across the NHS. It hopes to encourage doctors and other staff to report 'near-misses' when things almost go wrong. The change of emphasis is away from the current blame culture and is more about 'how' than 'whom'.

Some NHS trusts are participating in patient safety training and are monitoring mistakes and near-misses in order to learn how errors occur and how to set up systems to prevent them happening. An example of this was the Royal College of Anaesthetists' edict that nitrous oxide gas should not be included in the same anaesthetic equipment as oxygen in order to avoid accidental administration in an emergency.

USING LICENSED DRUGS FOR UNLICENSED PURPOSES

The efficacy of each drug is tested in clinical trials. When these are completed, the drug is licensed to be used for specific conditions. These conditions are outlined in the data sheet or Summary of Product Characteristics (SPC) for the drug, along with the doses and any contraindications that may apply and the side-effects of the drug. The data sheet will also outline any monitoring required. In the case of clozapine, the company also has to provide the monitoring of white blood cells, which are at risk because of the drug. Product licences for generic drugs may differ between manufacturers.

If a product is used within the product licence and a patient suffers from a serious side-effect, they may sue for any damage sustained (strict liability). If a medicine is used outside the product licence, then the clinician must be able to justify such use and to show documentation of any necessary investigations. Usage outside the product licence is common in certain areas, particularly in paediatrics, as most medicines are licensed only for use in adults. Some Trusts now have a mechanism for logging non-licensed use of new drugs. Some Trusts also have their own forms that need to be completed and placed in the patient's case notes to record the decision-making process in these circumstances; if such a form does not exist, then the decision should still be recorded in the case notes, together with a statement to the effect that the patient has been informed.

CLINICAL TRIALS

Trials are carried out on all new drugs at each stage of their development, for various reasons. The trials with which clinicians are most familiar are in phase three of development, just before the licence application is prepared. The results of these trials will establish the drug's place in therapy of the relevant disease. They will provide further knowledge on side effects, drug interactions and doses for specific patient groups.

If a manufacturer is organizing the trial, then it should ensure that the clinical trial certificate exemption has been obtained from the licensing authority and should inform the clinician that this has been done. If a manufacturer is not involved, then the local research ethics committee (LREC) can advise on what is needed. For a trial involving several centres, the manufacturer will obtain overall ethics approval, but each centre will need to gain approval from its local ethics committee.

The trial itself can take a number of forms. An open study is one in which both the clinician and the patient know what is being taken. Usually, this will be the active drug. The purpose of such a study will be to obtain further information on the drug, e.g. side-effects or the effects of long-term use.

In a single-blind study, the clinician will know what is being taken but the patient will not know which option has been assigned to them. These studies usually compare one or more doses of the drug being tested with a placebo. Sometimes there are clinical or ethical reasons that mean a placebo cannot be used, so the new drug will be compared with an existing one that is known to be efficacious in the same disease.

In a double-blind study, the substances used are the same as for a single-blind study, but the clinician is also unaware of which drug has been assigned to which patient, i.e. both the clinician and the patient are 'blinded'. This eliminates bias if the clinician is involved in assessing the patient's response to a given drug. Blindness can be lost if there are certain side-effects; in this case, the manufacturer may suggest that two clinicians be involved: one to administer the medication and the other to assess the patient's symptoms.

The outward appearance of both agents (active drug and placebo, or two drugs being compared with each other) should be the same; if this is not possible, then each person should have two tablets – one active, the other inactive. This is known as a 'double dummy'.

In certain situations, such as severe depression or epilepsy, it may not be ethically acceptable to leave a patient on only placebo or to use a comparison with an existing drug. This problem may be overcome by giving the new drug or placebo in addition to an established therapy. This is called an 'add-on study'.

The trial has to continue for as long as it takes the treatment to work. In the case of depression, it would be unrealistic to expect a full effect in less than three weeks.

If the trial is comparing two drugs, then it should use equivalent doses of both drugs, e.g. in the comparison of painkillers, it would be unreasonable to compare a single daily dose of aspirin with two paracetamol tablets taken four times a day.

In testing a new drug, the number of patients being treated should be enough for any difference to be seen clearly, i.e. the study needs to be powered sufficiently (in the statistical sense). This minimum number required will vary according to the condition being treated. However, for clinical reasons, it is sometimes useful to run a trial involving just one patient (an '$n = 1$ trial'). The patient will be asked to use one treatment for a period of time and then to use another treatment or placebo for a similar time. The response during each phase is monitored.

The following classification of clinical trials is used by the pharmaceutical industry:

- Phase I trial: clinical pharmacology and toxicity.
- Phase II trial: initial clinical investigation.
- Phase III trial: full-scale treatment evaluation.
- Phase IV trial: post-marketing surveillance.

LOCAL RESEARCH ETHICS COMMITTEES

This is found in HSG (19) 5, which states that each health area should have an LREC to advise NHS bodies on the ethical acceptability of research proposals involving human subjects.

Membership

An LREC should have 8–12 members to allow for a sufficiently broad range of experience and expertise, so that the scientific and medical aspects of a research project can be reconciled with the welfare of the research subjects and any broader ethical implications. It is suggested that members be drawn from a wide range of people, including:

- hospital medical staff
- nursing staff
- general practitioners
- two or more laypeople.

Legal aspects

On 1 May 2004, a change took place in European law governing clinical trials, which changed the legal framework for clinical trials on medicinal products. These regulations, the EU Clinical Trials Directive 2001/20, were implemented through the Medicines for Human Use (Clinical Trials) Regulations 2004. Following detailed discussion, Universities UK and the Department of Health reassured universities and NHS bodies that the regulations did not change the underlying allocation and responsibilities and potential liabilities in collaborative academic trials.

Universities have insurance cover for negligent harm. NHS bodies take on liability for clinical negligence that harms individuals towards whom the NHS has a duty of care. The policy of NHS indemnity for clinical trials conducted with NHS permission continues to apply. From April 2004, research-active NHS bodies have had to comply with a controls-assurance standard for research governance and to report compliance as part of NHS-wide arrangements for clinical and financial risk management. If a clinical trial involves an NHS body's employees or otherwise affects its duty of care, then its permission is required before the trial commences at that site; these arrangements reduce the risk (to the NHS and to university employers of medical academic staff) of unauthorized clinical research resulting in unexpected liabilities.

Under UK regulations, there is a legal requirement for ethical review, providing a mechanism to ensure that the trial design respects the dignity, rights, safety and wellbeing of participants. Ethical review also ensures that the information provided when seeking consent is sufficient to convey an understanding of the risks. The process leading to a Clinical Trial Authorization should provide an assurance that the protocol takes account of known risks associated with the medicines under investigation. It also confirms that there are arrangements for the allocation or delegation of all the legal responsibilities relating to the initiation and management of the trial, and to pharmacovigilance.

PATIENT GROUP DIRECTIONS (ENGLAND ONLY)

These are described in HSC 2000/026, which replaces HSC 1998/051, entitled *A Report on the Supply and Administration of Medicines under Group Protocols*. They allow a medicine to be supplied for a patient by a specific health professional without a prescription written by a doctor. The professional involved must work to a protocol drawn up by a doctor or dentist, a senior pharmacist, and a member of the profession who will be giving the supply to the patient. Only named individuals can make the supply, and they must be trained in the application of the protocol.

The largest patient group direction at the moment has concerned pharmacists in some health authorities who have supplied emergency hormonal contraception from retail pharmacy by this means. Day-surgery units have also found the mechanism useful, when standard antibiotic cover or analgesia to take home is used in specific procedures.

SUPPLEMENTARY PRESCRIBING

Non-medical Professionals may now train to be supplementary prescribers. Once qualified, they may then write prescriptions for a patient after the patient has been assessed and diagnosed by their doctor (the Independent Prescriber).

Supplementary prescribing must follow a Clinical Management Plan drawn up for the patient. The Independent Prescriber may therefore limit e.g. the dose range to be used by the Supplementary Prescriber.

The full criteria for the scheme are on www.doh.gov.uk/supplementary prescribing. This scheme would lend itself to the management of therapy with Lithium or Clozapine, so that the doctor can see the patient at intervals dictated by clinical need, with intermediate dose adjustments being made by the Supplementary Prescriber. The Trust must be involved with the setting up of the scheme, and only personnel trained and registered for the role may work in this way.

REFERENCE

Department of Health (2004). Report maps road to medication safety. *CMO Update* **38**, 2.

8

Professional liability and negligence

EU LAW AND MEDICAL QUALIFICATIONS

Free movement of people in the EU

In principle, the free movement of people, including medical professionals, between member countries of the European Union (EU) is envisaged by the Treaty of Rome. Indeed, the European Court has stated that:

> … the provisions of the Treaty [of Rome] relating to freedom of movement of persons are intended to facilitate the pursuit by [European] Community citizens of occupational activities of all kinds throughout the Community, and to preclude measures which might place Community citizens at a disadvantage when they wish to pursue an economic activity in the territory of another Member State.

In practice, however, there have been cases in which the European Court has upheld the effects of barriers to cross-border activity related to the different ways in which member states organize and regulate certain professions.

Mutual recognition of qualifications

On the one hand, the principle of subsidiarity (Article 5 of the Treaty) tends to protect the right of member countries of the EU to organize and regulate professions. On the other hand, in the case of professions such as those relating to medicine and allied disciplines, sectoral Directives (Article 47 of the Treaty, as amended by the Amsterdam Treaty) tend towards the mutual recognition of professional qualifications between member countries in order to achieve non-discrimination of professionals on the basis of nationality:

(1) In order to make it easier for persons to take up and pursue activities as self-employed persons, the Council shall, acting in accordance with the procedure referred to in Article 251, issue directives for the mutual recognition of diplomas, certificates and other evidence of formal qualifications.

(2) For the same purpose, the Council shall, acting in accordance with the procedure referred to in Article 251, issue directives for the co-ordination of the provisions laid down by law, regulation or

administrative action in Member States concerning the taking-up and pursuit of activities of self-employed persons. The Council, acting unanimously throughout the procedure referred to in Article 251, shall decide on directives the implementation of which involves in at least one Member State amendment of the existing principles laid down by law governing the professions with respect to training and conditions of access for natural persons. In other cases the Council shall act by qualified majority.

(3) In the case of the medical and allied and pharmaceutical professions, the progressive abolition of restrictions shall be dependent upon co-ordination of the conditions for their exercise in the various Member States.

Groups of medical and allied and pharmaceutical professions for which sectoral Directives exist include:

- doctors (specialists)
- doctors (general practitioners, GPs)
- nurses (general care)
- dentists
- midwives
- veterinary surgeons
- pharmacists.

There are two stages to the operation of the sectoral Directives. First, the training of these professions is coordinated between member countries. Second, mutual recognition of the corresponding professional qualifications takes place.

In the UK, the recognition of medical qualifications to allow a doctor to practise medicine is the remit of the General Medical Council (GMC). Currently, the GMC gives the following guidance on registration:

The process for gaining registration generally depends on the country where you obtained your primary medical qualification and your nationality. There are four main groups of doctors for the purposes of registration. The registration processes are different for each group:

- doctors qualifying from a UK medical school are eligible for provisional and full registration.
- doctors qualifying in another EEA Member State and who are nationals of an EEA Member State (or non-EEA nationals with European Community (EC) rights) are eligible for full registration. They are also eligible to apply for provisional registration if their medical education includes a period of postgraduate clinical training (sometimes referred to as internship training). The EEA includes the following countries: Austria, Belgium, Denmark, Finland, France, Germany, Greece, Iceland, Republic of Ireland, Italy, Liechtenstein, Luxembourg, Netherlands, Norway, Portugal, Spain and Sweden. Since 1 June 2002, doctors qualifying in Switzerland and who are EEA nationals (or non-EEA nationals with EC rights) or Swiss nationals are also eligible for full registration. This also applies to Swiss nationals who have qualified in another EEA Member State.

- doctors qualifying in the following countries: Australia, Hong Kong, Malaysia (if the degrees awarded by the University of Malaya are granted on or before 31 December 1989), New Zealand, Singapore, South Africa and the West Indies may be eligible for provisional and full registration.
- doctors who qualify in other countries not listed above may be eligible for limited and full registration. These include non-EEA nationals who do not benefit under EC law who have qualified in another EEA Member State.
- EEA nationals (and non-EEA nationals with EC rights) who qualify in other countries not listed above may be eligible for provisional or full registration if they have practised medicine in another EEA Member State.

CONTRACTUAL LIABILITY FOR SERVICE PROVISION

The law of contract

A contract is an agreement that can be enforced by law. Note that while all contracts are agreements, an agreement is not necessarily a contract. The characteristic components of a contract are as follows:

- offer
- acceptance
- consideration
- intention
- capacity.

Breach of contract

A doctor cannot be expected, under law, to guarantee success; for example, a proposed course of treatment might fail in spite of the best efforts of the medical profession. Thus, depending on the terms of the contract, liability may not normally be imposed on a doctor purely on the basis of failing to achieve an intended clinical goal. In order for this to be the case, the doctor (or clinical team) must exercise reasonable care and skill. Under Section 13 of the **Supply of Goods and Services Act 1982**:

> In a contract for the supply of a service where the supplier is acting in the course of a business, there is an implied term that the supplier will carry out the service with reasonable care and skill.

Tort

Central to medical profession liability is tort. This is a civil wrong, other than a breach of contract, which gives the right to bring an action in a civil court. (Such actions might include nuisance, negligence, defamation and trespass.)

Two key points to bear in mind are (i) that the legal responsibility of a UK-based hospital doctor is to the health authority or the National Health Service (NHS) Trust in which they work, and (ii) that a NHS patient can only sue in tort.

BREACH OF DUTY OF CONFIDENTIALITY

A doctor has a duty of confidentiality towards his or her patients. Information about a patient is confidential not only during the time that the doctor is treating the patient but also after the end of such treatment. Under certain circumstances, however, it is justifiable to breach confidentiality. The prime confidentiality obligations now derive from Data Protection Act and Human Rights Act provisions.

Royal College of Psychiatrists guidance on confidentiality

The Royal College of Psychiatrists (2000) has issued the following guidance on confidentiality in relation to psychiatric patients:

> Good psychiatric practice starts from the premise that all information about the patient is confidential. However, there are many conflicting demands, including issues of public safety, the importance of involving relatives and carers, and the sharing of information between the police, courts and agencies responsible for child protection.

> To achieve this the psychiatrist will:

> - treat information about patients as confidential
> - be familiar with the recommendations of the Caldicott report, and seek the advice of the Caldicott guardian where issues of breaches of confidentiality are raised
> - communicate high-quality and correct clinical information to members of clinical teams
> - communicate across agencies according to agreed protocols and practice
> - communicate fully with general practitioners and with the expectation that the communication will be confidential
> - work to achieve good communication between patients and their family/carers where possible
> - respect the confidentiality of sensitive third-party information and only divulge such information either to the patient or others with the consent of that party
> - ensure the use of identifiable information relating to persons suffering from psychiatric disorder for use in research and audit is governed by the protocols of the local ethics committee
> - use non-identifiable information to inform service development, commissioning and performance monitoring

- be aware of the need to share information beyond the immediate clinical team and health care practitioners on the rare occasions where a person with severe psychiatric disorder poses a threat to others or self
- be cognisant of the information needs of informal carers about persons suffering from severe mental illness
- be aware of the needs of children, and the responsibilities imposed on health care professionals by the Children Acts
- always consult with local child protection officers where the child is placed at possible short- or long-term risk
- be familiar with the GMC's guidance on confidentiality.

Examples of unacceptable practice include:

- failing to pay sufficient attention to the importance of confidentiality
- failing to provide appropriate information where necessary
- inappropriately providing confidential information.

Note that there is also guidance on confidentiality from the Department of Health (2004).

Justified disclosure of patient information

The GMC (2004) has issued the following guidance in relation to circumstances in which it is appropriate to disclose confidential patient information:

SECTION 3 DISCLOSURE OF INFORMATION

SHARING INFORMATION WITH OTHERS PROVIDING CARE

7. Where patients have consented to treatment, express consent is not usually needed before relevant personal information is shared to enable the treatment to be provided. For example, express consent would not be needed before general practitioners disclose relevant personal information so that a medical secretary can type a referral letter. Similarly, where a patient has agreed to be referred for an X-ray physicians may make relevant information available to radiologists when requesting an X-ray. Doctors cannot treat patients safely, nor provide the continuity of care, without having relevant information about the patient's condition and medical history.

8. You should make sure that patients are aware that personal information about them will be shared within the health care team, unless they object, and of the reasons for this. It is particularly important to check that patients understand what will be disclosed if it is necessary to share personal information with anyone employed by another organisation or agency providing health or social care. You must respect the wishes of any patient who objects to particular information being shared with others providing care, except where this would put others at risk of death or serious harm.

9. You must make sure that anyone to whom you disclose personal information understands that it is given to them in confidence, which they must respect. Anyone receiving personal information in order to provide care is bound by a legal duty of confidence, whether or not they have contractual or professional obligations to protect confidentiality.

10. Circumstances may arise where a patient cannot be informed about the sharing of information, for example because of a medical emergency. In these cases you should pass relevant information promptly to those providing the patient's care.

SECTION 4 DISCLOSURE OF INFORMATION OTHER THAN FOR TREATMENT OF THE INDIVIDUAL PATIENT

PRINCIPLES

11. Information about patients is requested for a wide variety of purposes including education, research, monitoring and epidemiology, public health surveillance, clinical audit, administration and planning. You have a duty to protect patients' privacy and respect their autonomy. When asked to provide information you should
    a. Seek patients' consent to disclosure of any information wherever possible, whether or not you judge that patients can be identified from the disclosure.
    b. Anonymise data where unidentifiable data will serve the purpose.
    c. Keep disclosures to the minimum necessary.

12. The paragraphs which follow deal with obtaining consent, and what to do where consent is unobtainable, or it is impracticable to seek consent.

OBTAINING CONSENT

13. Seeking patients' consent to disclosure is part of good communication between doctors and patients, and is an essential part of respect for patients' autonomy and privacy.

CONSENT WHERE DISCLOSURES WILL HAVE PERSONAL CONSEQUENCES FOR PATIENTS

14. You must obtain express consent where patients may be personally affected by the disclosure, for example when disclosing personal information to a patient's employer. When seeking express consent you must make sure that patients are given enough information on which to base their decision, the reasons for the disclosure and the likely consequences of the disclosure. You should also explain how much information will be disclosed and to whom it will be given. If the patient withholds consent, or consent cannot be obtained, disclosures may be made only where they can be justified in the

public interest, usually where disclosure is essential to protect the patient, or someone else, from risk of death or serious harm.

CONSENT WHERE THE DISCLOSURE IS UNLIKELY TO HAVE PERSONAL CONSEQUENCES FOR PATIENTS

15. Disclosure of information about patients for purposes such as epidemiology, public health safety, or the administration of health services, or for use in education or training, clinical or medical audit, or research is unlikely to have personal consequences for the patient. In these circumstances you should still obtain patients' express consent to the use of identifiable data or arrange for members of the health care team to anonymise records (see also paragraphs 16 and 18).

16. However, where information is needed for the purposes of the kind set out in paragraph 15, and you are satisfied that it is not practicable either to obtain express consent to disclosure, nor for a member of the health care team to anonymise records, data may be disclosed without express consent. Usually such disclosures will be made to allow a person outside the health care team to anonymise the records. Only where it is essential for the purpose may identifiable records be disclosed. Such disclosures must be kept to the minimum necessary for the purpose. In all such cases you must be satisfied that patients have been told, or have had access to written material informing them:

    a. That their records may be disclosed to persons outside the team which provided their care.

    b. Of the purpose and extent of the disclosure, for example, to produce anonymised data for use in education, administration, research or audit.

    c. That the person given access to records will be subject to a duty of confidentiality.

    d. That they have a right to object to such a process, and that their objection will be respected, except where the disclosure is essential to protect the patient, or someone else, from risk of death or serious harm.

17. Where you have control of personal information about patients, you must not allow anyone access to them for the purposes of the kind set out in paragraph 15, unless the person has been properly trained and authorised by the health authority, NHS trust or comparable body and is subject to a duty of confidentiality in their employment or because of their registration with a statutory regulatory body.

DISCLOSURES IN THE PUBLIC INTEREST

18. In cases where you have considered all the available means of obtaining consent, but you are satisfied that it is not practicable to do so, or that patients are not competent to give consent, or exceptionally, in cases where patients withhold consent, personal information may be disclosed in the public interest where the benefits

to an individual or to society of the disclosure outweigh the public and the patient's interest in keeping the information confidential.

19. In all such cases you must weigh the possible harm (both to the patient, and the overall trust between doctors and patients) against the benefits which are likely to arise from the release of information.

20. Ultimately, the 'public interest' can be determined only by the courts; but the GMC may also require you to justify your actions if we receive a complaint about the disclosure of personal information without a patient's consent.

SECTION 5 PUTTING THE PRINCIPLES INTO PRACTICE

DISCLOSURES WHICH BENEFIT PATIENTS INDIRECTLY

MONITORING PUBLIC HEALTH AND THE SAFETY OF MEDICINES AND DEVICES INCLUDING DISCLOSURES TO CANCER AND OTHER REGISTRIES

22. Professional organisations and government regulatory bodies which monitor the public health or the safety of medicines or devices, as well as cancer and other registries, rely on information from patients' records for their effectiveness in safeguarding the public health. For example, the effectiveness of the yellow card scheme run by the Committee on Safety of Medicines depends on information provided by clinicians. You must co-operate by providing relevant information wherever possible. The notification of some communicable diseases is required by law (see also paragraph 43), and in other cases you should provide information in anonymised form, wherever that would be sufficient.

23. Where personal information is needed, you should seek express consent before disclosing information, whenever that is practicable. For example, where patients are receiving treatment there will usually be an opportunity for a health care professional to discuss disclosure of information with them.

24. Personal information may sometimes be sought about patients with whom health care professionals are not in regular contact. Doctors should therefore make sure that patients are given information about the possible value of their data in protecting the public health in the longer-term, at the initial consultation or at another suitable occasion when they attend a surgery or clinic. Patients should be given the information set out in paragraph 16: it should be clear that they may object to disclosures at any point. You must record any objections so that patients' wishes can be respected. In such cases, you may pass on anonymised information if asked to do so.

25. Where patients have not expressed an objection, you should assess the likely benefit of the disclosure to the public and commitment to confidentiality of the organisation requesting the information. If there is little or no evident public benefit, you should not disclose information without the express consent of the patient.

26. Where it is not practicable to seek patients' consent for disclosure of personal information for these purposes, or where patients are not competent to give consent, you must consider whether disclosures would be justified in the public interest, by weighing the benefits to the public health of the disclosure against the possible detriment to the patient.

27. The automatic transfer of personal information to a registry, whether by electronic or other means, before informing the patient that information will be passed on, is unacceptable save in the most exceptional circumstances. These would be where a court has already decided that there is such an overwhelming public interest in the disclosure of information to a registry that patients' rights to confidentiality are overridden; or where you are willing and able to justify the disclosure, potentially before a court or to the GMC, on the same grounds.

CLINICAL AUDIT AND EDUCATION

28. Anonymised data will usually be sufficient for clinical audit and for education. When anonymising records you should follow the guidance on obtaining consent in paragraphs 15–17 above. You should not disclose non-anonymised data for clinical audit or education without the patient's consent.

ADMINISTRATION AND FINANCIAL AUDIT

29. You should record financial or other administrative data separately from clinical information, and provide it in anonymised form, wherever that is possible.

30. Decisions about the disclosure of clinical records for administrative or financial audit purposes, for example where health authority staff seek access to patients' records as part of the arrangements for verifying NHS payments, are unlikely to bring your registration into question, provided that, before allowing access to patients' records, you follow the guidance in paragraphs 15–17. Only the relevant part of the record should be made available for scrutiny.

MEDICAL RESEARCH

31. Where research projects depend on using identifiable information or samples, and it is not practicable to contact patients to seek their consent, this fact should be drawn to the attention of a research ethics committee so that it can consider whether the likely benefits of the research outweigh the loss of confidentiality. Disclosures may otherwise be improper, even if the recipients of the information are registered medical practitioners. The decision of a research ethics committee would be taken into account by a court if a claim for breach of confidentiality were made, but the court's judgement would be based on its own assessment of whether the public interest was served. More detailed guidance is issued by the medical royal colleges and other bodies.

PUBLICATION OF CASE-HISTORIES AND PHOTOGRAPHS

32. You must obtain express consent from patients before publishing personal information about them as individuals in media to which the public has access, for example in journals or text books, whether or not you believe the patient can be identified. Express consent must therefore be sought to the publication of, for example, case-histories about, or photographs of, patients. Where you wish to publish information about a patient who has died, you should take into account the guidance in paragraphs 40–41 before deciding whether or not to do so.

DISCLOSURES WHERE DOCTORS HAVE DUAL RESPONSIBILITIES

33. Situations arise where doctors have contractual obligations to third parties, such as companies or organisations, as well as obligations to patients. Such situations occur, for example, when doctors:
    a. Provide occupational health services or medical care for employees of a company or organisation.
    b. Are employed by an organisation such as an insurance company.
    c. Work for an agency assessing claims for benefits.
    d. Provide medical care for patients and are subsequently asked to provide medical reports or information for third parties about them.
    e. Work as police surgeons.
    f. Work in the armed forces.
    g. Work in the prison service.
34. If you are asked to write a report about and/or examine a patient, or to disclose information from existing records for a third party to whom you have contractual obligations, you must:
    a. Be satisfied that the patient has been told at the earliest opportunity about the purpose of the examination and/or disclosure, the extent of the information to be disclosed and the fact that relevant information cannot be concealed or withheld. You might wish to show the form to the patient before you complete it to ensure the patient understands the scope of the information requested.
    b. Obtain, or have seen, written consent to the disclosure from the patient or a person properly authorised to act on the patient's behalf. You may, however, accept written assurances from an officer of a government department that the patient's written consent has been given.
    c. Disclose only information relevant to the request for disclosure: accordingly, you should not usually disclose the whole record. The full record may be relevant to some benefits paid by government departments.
    d. Include only factual information you can substantiate, presented in an unbiased manner.
    e. The Access to Medical Reports Act 1988 entitles patients to see reports written about them before they are disclosed, in some

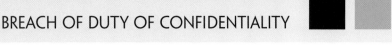
circumstances. In all circumstances you should check whether patients wish to see their report, unless patients have clearly and specifically stated that they do not wish to do so.

35. Disclosures without consent to employers, insurance companies, or any other third party, can be justified only in exceptional circumstances, for example, when they are necessary to protect others from risk of death or serious harm.

DISCLOSURES TO PROTECT THE PATIENT OR OTHERS

36. Disclosure of personal information without consent may be justified where failure to do so may expose the patient or others to risk of death or serious harm. Where third parties are exposed to a risk so serious that it outweighs the patient's privacy interest, you should seek consent to disclosure where practicable. If it is not practicable, you should disclose information promptly to an appropriate person or authority. You should generally inform the patient before disclosing the information.

37. Such circumstances may arise, for example:
    a. Where a colleague, who is also a patient, is placing patients at risk as a result of illness or other medical condition. If you are in doubt about whether disclosure is justified you should consult an experienced colleague, or seek advice from a professional organisation. The safety of patients must come first at all times …
    b. Where a patient continues to drive, against medical advice, when unfit to do so. In such circumstances you should disclose relevant information to the medical adviser of the Driver and Vehicle Licensing Agency without delay …
    c. Where a disclosure may assist in the prevention or detection of a serious crime. Serious crimes, in this context, will put someone at risk of death or serious harm, and will usually be crimes against the person, such as abuse of children.

CHILDREN AND OTHER PATIENTS WHO MAY LACK COMPETENCE TO GIVE CONSENT

38. Problems may arise if you consider that a patient is incapable of giving consent to treatment or disclosure because of immaturity, illness or mental incapacity. If such patients ask you not to disclose information to a third party, you should try to persuade them to allow an appropriate person to be involved in the consultation. If they refuse and you are convinced that it is essential, in their medical interests, you may disclose relevant information to an appropriate person or authority. In such cases you must tell the patient before disclosing any information, and, where appropriate, seek and carefully consider the views of an advocate or carer. You should document in the patient's record the steps you have taken to obtain consent and the reasons for deciding to disclose information.

39. If you believe a patient to be a victim of neglect or physical, sexual or emotional abuse and that the patient cannot give or withhold consent to disclosure, you should give information promptly to an appropriate responsible person or statutory agency, where you believe that the disclosure is in the patient's best interests. You should usually inform the patient that you intend to disclose the information before doing so. Such circumstances may arise in relation to children, where concerns about possible abuse need to be shared with other agencies such as social services. Where appropriate you should inform those with parental responsibility about the disclosure. If, for any reason, you believe that disclosure of information is not in the best interests of an abused or neglected patient, you must still be prepared to justify your decision.

DISCLOSURE AFTER A PATIENT'S DEATH

40. You still have an obligation to keep personal information confidential after a patient dies. The extent to which confidential information may be disclosed after a patient's death will depend on the circumstances. These include the nature of the information, whether that information is already public knowledge or can be anonymised, and the intended use to which the information will be put. You should also consider whether the disclosure of information may cause distress to, or be of benefit to, the patient's partner or family.

41. There are a number of circumstances in which you may be asked to disclose, or wish to use, information about patients who have died. For example:

    a. To assist a Coroner, Procurator Fiscal or other similar officer in connection with an inquest or fatal accident inquiry. In these circumstances you should provide relevant information …

    b. As part of National Confidential Enquiries or other clinical audit or for education or research. The publication of properly anonymised case studies would be unlikely to be improper in these contexts.

    c. On death certificates. The law requires you to complete death certificates honestly and fully.

    d. To obtain information relating to public health surveillance. Anonymised information should be used unless identifiable data is essential to the study.

42. Particular difficulties may arise when there is a conflict of interest between parties affected by the patient's death. For example, if an insurance company seeks information in order to decide whether to make a payment under a life assurance policy, you should release information in accordance with the requirements of the Access to Health Records Act 1990 or with the authorisation of those lawfully entitled to deal with the person's estate who have been fully informed of the consequences of disclosure. It may also be appropriate to inform those close to the patient.

SECTION 6 DISCLOSURE IN CONNECTION WITH JUDICIAL OR OTHER STATUTORY PROCEEDINGS

43. You must disclose information to satisfy a specific statutory requirement, such as notification of a known or suspected communicable disease.

44. You must also disclose information if ordered to do so by a judge or presiding officer of a court. You should object to the judge or the presiding officer if attempts are made to compel you to disclose what appear to you to be irrelevant matters, for example matters relating to relatives or partners of the patient, who are not parties to the proceedings.

45. You should not disclose personal information to a third party such as a solicitor, police officer or officer of a court without the patient's express consent, except in the circumstances described at paragraphs 36–37, 39 and 41.

46. You may disclose personal information in response to an official request from a statutory regulatory body for any of the health care professions, where that body determines that this is necessary in the interests of justice and for the safety of other patients. Wherever practicable you should discuss this with the patient. There may be exceptional cases where, even though the patient objects, disclosure is justified.

If you decide to disclose confidential information you must be prepared to explain and justify your decision.

Disclosure in the public interest: the *Egdell* case

In respect of the issue of disclosure in the public interest, the case of *W* v. *Egdell* (1990) is of importance in relation to the balancing act between patient confidentiality and competing public interests.

Patient W suffered from schizophrenia and was detained in a secure unit under a restriction order made under Section 60 and Section 65 of the Mental Health Act 1959. He had been convicted of the manslaughter of five people and had also wounded two others. He subsequently exercised his right, under Section 41 of the Mental Health Act 1983, to apply for review by a Mental Health Review Tribunal for discharge (or transfer with a view to discharge). The responsible medical officer (RMO) for W was of the opinion that the patient's schizophrenic symptomatology could be controlled adequately by pharmacotherapy and supported his application. W's solicitors instructed Dr Egdell, another psychiatrist, to review W and prepare a report on him. This report was unfavourable to W and recommended against the patient being transferred from the secure unit. In his report, Dr Egdell suggested that W had an abnormal, possibly psychopathic, personality. Dr Egdell expressed concern about the fact that the patient had an interest in what he (the patient) referred to as 'fireworks', by which he meant explosive devices (pipes filled with explosives). On reading Dr Egdell's report, W's solicitors withdrew the application to the Mental Health

Review Tribunal. Dr Egdell asked that a copy of his report be included in W's hospital records, but this was refused by W's solicitors. Dr Egdell then disclosed a copy of his report to the medical director of the hospital in which W was a patient, and in due course the Home Office also received a copy.

The case came up for review again, this time under Section 67 of the Mental Health Act 1983. Although W's solicitors obtained an injunction barring Dr Egdell from disclosing his report at the hearing, the Home Secretary was able to put forward information gathered by Dr Egdell. As a result, W brought actions in equity and contract against Dr Egdell, alleging a breach of duty of confidence.

At trial, the issue of concern was not whether Dr Egdell was under a duty of confidence – for it was clear that he was. Rather,

> The question is as to the breadth of that duty. Did the duty extend so far as to bar disclosure to the medical director of the hospital? Did it bar disclosure to the Home Office?

The Court of Appeal ruled that, in this case, the public interest of the protection and safety to the public was greater than the public interest in maintaining confidence.

NEGLIGENCE

Close and direct proximity

A duty of care is owed by a medical professional to his or her patient and to those in 'close proximity' to the patient, i.e. the immediate family of the patient. It has not yet been determined in case law, however, how 'close' a relative needs to be in order to be owed a duty of care by the patient's doctor. Also, a person in close proximity does not necessarily have to be a relative; again, this area of the law remains uncertain and difficult.

Duty of care

Line of duty of care

The legal duty of medical care to a patient may be considered to have a linear form, beginning with the presentation, in some manner, of a person requiring some form of care and ending with completion of the relevant treatment(s).

Time of initial establishment

At present, case law does not give definitive guidance on the exact time of commencement of the legal duty of care. (It may be considered, variously, to arise when a patient first enters a hospital building or general practice surgery, when a patient first formally presents to a doctor for clinical interview and examination, or when a patient formally agrees to a particular course of treatment, for example.)

Secretary of State for Health

Under Section 1 of the **National Health Service Act 1977**, the Secretary of State for Health has a duty

> ... to continue the promotion in England and Wales of a comprehensive health service designed to secure improvement (a) in the physical and mental health of the people of those countries, and (b) in the prevention, diagnosis and treatment of illness, and for that purpose to provide or secure the effective provision of services in accordance with this Act.

More specifically, these duties are listed in Section 3 of this Act, as follows.

> It is the Secretary of State's duty to provide to such an extent as he considers necessary to meet all reasonable requirements –
>
> (a) hospital accommodation;
> (b) other accommodation for the purpose of any service provided under this Act;
> (c) medical, dental, nursing and ambulance services;
> (d) such other facilities for the care of expectant mothers and nursing mothers and young children as he considers are appropriate as part of the health service;
> (e) such facilities for the prevention of illness, the care of persons suffering from illness and the after-care of persons who have suffered from illness as he considers are appropriate as part of the health service;
> (f) such other services as are required for the diagnosis and treatment of illness.

Emergencies

Although a 'Good-Samaritan law' does not exist formally within English law, the GMC advises medical practitioners:

> In an emergency, wherever it may arise, you must offer anyone at risk the assistance you could reasonably be expected to provide.

It could be argued that English case law would tend to agree. For example, the judge in *Barnes* v. *Crabtree* (1955) stated:

> In a case of real acute emergency a doctor under the National Health Service scheme was under an obligation to treat any patient who was acutely ill; for example, if there was a motor accident and someone was lying seriously injured.

Breach of duty of care

Bolam test

In the case of *Bolam* v. *Friern Hospital Management Committee* (1957), a psychiatric patient was given electroconvulsive therapy (ECT) without the use of a muscle relaxant. In addition, apart from his lower jaw, which was controlled manually, there was no use of restraints. During this treatment, the patient sustained orthopaedic injuries (pelvic fractures and dislocation of the hip joints). The patient sued. At the time the patient had sustained these injuries, the issues of muscle relaxation, sedation and restraint during ECT were the subjects of debate within the medical profession, and no definitive protocol had been laid down in respect of these. The patient lost his case. Having established that there exists the 'man on the Clapham omnibus', who is not a highly trained medical specialist, the case held that:

> ... where you get a situation which involves the use of some special skill or competence, then the test of whether there has been negligence or not is not the test of the man on the Clapham omnibus, because he has not got this special skill. The test is the standard of the ordinary skilled man exercising and professing to exercise that special skill. A man need not possess the highest skill at the risk of being found negligent. It is well-established law that is sufficient if he exercises the ordinary skill of an ordinary man exercising that particular act ... A doctor is not guilty of negligence if he has acted in accordance with a practice accepted as proper by a responsible body of medical opinion of medical men skilled in that particular act.

This is the *Bolam* test, and it is central in cases of alleged professional negligence; it should be noted that the *Bolam* test has been considered in subsequent cases (such as Bolitho). Note that the 'practice accepted as proper by a responsible body of medical opinion of medical men skilled in that particular act' refers to the accepted practice at the material time, and not to accepted practice at the later time of a trial, by when it may have changed owing to advances in medicine, for example. Also, in the case of medical specialties, the medical doctors 'skilled in that particular act' should be taken as referring to a doctor exercising the ordinary skills of their speciality (see *Maynard* v. *West Midlands Regional Health Authority* (1984)).

PROFESSIONAL LIABILITY

So far as the medical profession is concerned, medical professional liability may be attached to a person correctly designated a 'registered medical practitioner' or to a person who makes a false declaration that they are qualified as a 'registered medical practitioner'; in the latter case, criminal liability also attaches.

Registered medical practitioner

Under Section 3 of the Medical Act 1983:

> Subject to the provisions of this Act any person who

> (a) holds one or more primary United Kingdom qualifications and has passed a qualifying examination and satisfied the requirements of this Part of this Act as to experience; or

(b) being a national of any member State of the Communities, holds one or more primary European qualifications;

is entitled to be registered under this section as a fully registered medical practitioner.

The current guidance on registration issued by the GMC is given earlier in this chapter.

False declaration of being medically qualified

Under Section 49 of the Medical Act 1983, anyone

… who wilfully and falsely pretends to be or takes or uses the name or title or physician, doctor of medicine, licentiate in medicine or surgery, bachelor of medicine, surgeon, general practitioner or apothecary, or any name, title, addition or description implying that he is registered under any provision of this Act, or that he is recognised by law as a physician or surgeon or licentiate in medicine and surgery or a practitioner in medicine or an apothecary, shall be liable on summary conviction to a fine.

Duty to keep up with professional developments

The GMC (2001) makes it clear that doctors have a duty to keep up with professional developments:

10. You must keep your knowledge and skills up to date throughout your working life. In particular, you should take part regularly in educational activities which maintain and further develop your competence and performance.
11. Some parts of medical practice are governed by law or are regulated by other statutory bodies. You must observe and keep up to date with the laws and statutory codes of practice which affect your work.

Other duties

The duty of care and the duty of confidence have been considered in earlier sections of this chapter. Other duties that have some backing in English case law include:

- the duty to write prescriptions clearly;
- the duty to protect patients from self-harm;
- the duty to protect patients from harming other people.

REFERENCES

Department of Health (2004). *Patient Confidentiality and Access to Health Records.* www.dh.gov.uk/PolicyAndGuidance/InformationTechnology/PatientConfiden tialityAndCaldicottGuardians/fs/en.

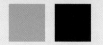

General Medical Council (2001). *Good Medical Practice*. London: General Medical Council.

General Medical Council (2004). *Confidentiality: Protecting and Providing Information*. London: General Medical Council.

Royal College of Psychiatrists (2000). *Good Psychiatric Practice*. London: Royal College of Psychiatrists.

9

Mental Health Review Tribunals

Mental Health Review Tribunals are covered in Part V (sections 65–79, inclusive) of the Mental Health Act.

CONSTITUTION AND RELATED ASPECTS

Although their establishment is provided for by Section 65 of the Mental Health Act 1983, Mental Health Review Tribunals are independent. Their membership is appointed by the Lord Chancellor.

There exists one Mental Health Review Tribunal for each National Health Service (NHS) Regional Health Authority in England, and one for Wales.

The Lord Chancellor appoints the following three types of members of Mental Health Review Tribunals:

- *Legal members:* appointed by the Lord Chancellor and having such legal experience as the Lord Chancellor considers suitable.
- *Medical members:* registered medical practitioners appointed by the Lord Chancellor after consultation with the Secretary of State.
- *Lay members:* appointed by the Lord Chancellor after consultation with the Secretary of State and having experience in administration, knowledge of social services or other qualifications or experience considered suitable by the Lord Chancellor.

The chair of each Mental Health Review Tribunal is a legal member appointed by the Lord Chancellor. In turn, the chair usually appoints the individual members of a given Mental Health Review Tribunal so that there is at least one legal member, one medical member, and one lay member, as defined above. Any three or more such members, constituted in this manner, may exercise the jurisdiction of a Mental Health Review Tribunal.

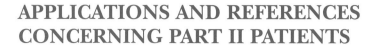

APPLICATIONS AND REFERENCES CONCERNING PART II PATIENTS

Applications to tribunals

Table 9.1 summarizes the sections of Part II of the Mental Health Act 1983 under which an application may be made to a Mental Health Review Tribunal, the period during which such application may be made (known as the relevant period), and by whom such application may be made.

TABLE 9.1 Access to Mental Health Review Tribunal

Section	Purpose of Section	Relevant period	By whom the application may be made
2	Admission for assessment	Within 14 days of admission	The patient
3	Admission for treatment	Within 6 months of admission	The patient
7	Reception into guardianship	Within 6 months of the application being accepted	The patient
16	Doctor reclassifies the mental disorder	Within 28 days of the applicant being informed that the report has been furnished	The patient; the nearest relative
19	Transfer from guardianship to hospital	Within 6 months of the patient being transferred	The patient
20	Duration of authority	The period for which authority for the patient's detention or guardianship is renewed by virtue of the report	The patient
25	Restriction of discharge by nearest relative	Within 28 days of the applicant being informed that the report has been furnished	The nearest relative
25A	Supervised aftercare	Within 6 months and then in each period	The patient; the nearest relative
29	Appointment of acting nearest relative by court	Within 12 months of the date of the order, and in any subsequent period of 12 months during which the order continues in force	The nearest relative

References to tribunals by Secretary of State

The Secretary of State may, at any time, refer to a Mental Health Review Tribunal the case of a patient who is liable to be detained or subject to guardianship under Part II of the Mental Health Act 1983. In order to furnish information for this purpose, any registered medical practitioner authorized by or on behalf of the

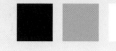
patient may, at any reasonable time, visit the patient, examine the patient in private, and require the production of and inspect any records relating to the detention or treatment of the patient in any hospital.

Duty of managers of hospitals to refer cases to tribunal

Provision is made for the automatic referral to a Mental Health Review Tribunal by hospital managers of the cases of patients detained under certain sections of Part II of the Mental Health Act 1983 when such patients have not exercised their right of such referral. This provides a safeguard against such patients being detained compulsorily for unduly long periods.

Section 3

If a patient admitted to hospital under Section 3 of the Mental Health Act 1983 (admission for treatment) has not exercised his or her right to apply to a Mental Health Review Tribunal, and if no application or reference has been made for the patient under any section of the Act, then the hospital manager must refer the patient's case to a Mental Health Review Tribunal at the end of the relevant period (six months).

Section 19

If a patient transferred from guardianship to hospital under Section 19 of the Mental Health Act 1983 (transfer from guardianship to hospital) has not exercised his or her right to apply to a Mental Health Review Tribunal, and if no application or reference has been made for the patient under any section of the Act, then the hospital manager must refer the patient's case to a Mental Health Review Tribunal at the end of the relevant period (six months).

Section 20

If the duration of authority for the detention of a patient in a hospital is renewed under Section 20 of the Mental Health Act 1983 (duration of authority), and a period of three years (or, in the case of a patient who has not reached 16 years of age, one year) has elapsed since his or her case was last considered by a Mental Health Review Tribunal, then the hospital manager must refer the patient's case to a Mental Health Review Tribunal.

Independent medical examination

In each of the above three cases (sections 3, 19 and 20), any registered medical practitioner authorized by or on behalf of the patient may, at any reasonable time, visit the patient, examine the patient in private, and require the production of and inspect any records relating to the detention or treatment of the patient in any hospital.

APPLICATIONS AND REFERENCES CONCERNING PART III PATIENTS

These are considered in Chapter 5.

DISCHARGE OF PATIENTS

Patients detained under Section 2

Under Section 72(1)(a) of the Mental Health Act 1983 (amended by Remedial Order 2001 in November 2001), a Mental Health Review Tribunal has the power to direct the discharge of a patient liable to be detained under Section 2 of the Act (admission for assessment) if the tribunal is not satisfied that:

- the patient is suffering from mental disorder or from mental disorder of a nature or degree that warrants his or her detention in hospital for assessment (or for assessment followed by treatment) for at least a limited period; or
- the detention of the patient is justified in the interests of his or her health or safety or with a view to the protection of others.

Patients detained under sections other than Section 2 and excluding restricted patients

Under Section 72(1)(b) of the Mental Health Act 1983 (Remedial) Order 2001, a Mental Health Review Tribunal has the power to direct the discharge of an unrestricted patient liable to be detained under a section of the Act other than Section 2 if the tribunal is not satisfied that:

- the patient is suffering from mental illness, psychopathic disorder, severe mental impairment or mental impairment or from any of those forms of disorder of a nature or degree that makes it appropriate for him or her to be liable to be detained in hospital for treatment; or
- it is necessary for the health or safety of the patient or for the protection of others that the patient should receive such treatment; or
- in the case of an application under Section 25 of the Act (restriction of discharge by nearest relative), the patient, if released, would be likely to act in a manner dangerous to others or to him- or herself.

The Mental Health Review Tribunal shall have regard:

- to the likelihood of medical treatment alleviating or preventing a deterioration of the patient's condition; and
- in the case of a patient suffering from mental illness or severe mental impairment, to the likelihood of the patient, if discharged, being able to care for him- or herself, to obtain the care needed or to guard against serious exploitation.

Delayed discharge

Rather than delay a decision in order to allow time for any necessary arrangements relating to discharge to be made (e.g. with respect to care or supervision in the community or accommodation), under Section 72(3) a Mental Health Review Tribunal may direct the discharge of a patient on a future date. Alternatively, the tribunal may:

■ with a view to facilitating the patient's discharge on a future date, recommend that the patient be granted leave of absence or transferred to another hospital or into guardianship; and
■ consider further the patient's case in the event of any such recommendation not being complied with.

Guardianship

Where application is made to a Mental Health Review Tribunal by or in respect of a patient who is subject to guardianship under the Mental Health Act 1983, under Section 72(4) the tribunal shall direct that the patient be discharged if they are satisfied that:

■ the patient is not suffering from mental illness, psychopathic disorder, severe mental impairment or mental impairment;
■ it is not necessary in the interests of the welfare of the patient, or for the protection of others, that the patient should remain under such guardianship.

Reclassification of form of mental disorder

Under Section 72(5), when a Mental Health Review Tribunal does not decide to discharge a patient, it may, if satisfied that the patient is suffering from a form of mental disorder other than that specified in the application, order or direction relating to the patient, direct that the classification of mental disorder in that application, order or direction be amended to one that appears more appropriate to the tribunal. For example, a patient may be reclassified from psychopathic disorder or severe mental impairment to mental impairment.

Restricted patients

Sections 73, 74 and 75 of the Mental Health Act 1983 deal with the power of Mental Health Review Tribunals to discharge restricted patients. The Secretary of State (in this case, the Home Secretary) has extended powers (compared with those of the Secretary of State in relation to Mental Health Review Tribunals assessing Part II patients) relating to the composition and proceedings of Mental Health Review Tribunals assessing restricted patients. These are not considered further here.

CODE OF PRACTICE

According to the Code of Practice (1989), Paragraph 14.12c:

There is a statutory obligation on the Managers to tell a detained patient of his right to apply to a mental health review tribunal. In addition, Managers should regard it as an obligation to ensure that patients and their nearest relatives know of the existence and role of these tribunals and of their respective rights of application to them. The Managers should ensure that patients remain aware of their rights to apply to a tribunal and are given every opportunity and assistance to exercise those rights, including facilities for representation. The patient should be told of his right to be represented by a lawyer of his choice, the Law Society's Mental Health Review Tribunal representation panel list and about other appropriate organisations, and should be given every assistance in using any of them. Managers should designate a member of staff to see personally every detained patient who applies to a tribunal or who is referred to a tribunal and to give them every reasonable assistance in securing representation (if the patient wishes).

SOCIAL CIRCUMSTANCES REPORTS

Gostin and Fennell (1992, p. 196) noted the crucial role of the social circumstances report for Mental Health Review Tribunals: 'A patient's social circumstances following his discharge from hospital are at the core of the tribunal's concerns.' They also commented: '… the tribunal cannot reach an informed decision … unless it has a clear picture of where and how a patient would live if he were to be discharged' (p. 200). If this information is not seen as sufficient when provided by the local authority, then the authors recommend seeking an independent social report.

Part B of Schedule 1 to the Mental Health Review Tribunal Rules 1983 sets out what is expected in reports (other than for conditionally discharged patients):

1. An up-to-date medical report, prepared for the tribunal, including the relevant medical history and a full report on the patient's mental condition.
2. An up-to-date social circumstances report, prepared for the tribunal including reports on the following
   (a) the patient's home and family circumstances, including the attitude of the patient's nearest relative or the person so acting;
   (b) the opportunities for employment or occupation and the housing facilities which would be available to the patient if discharged;
   (c) the availability of community support and the relevant medical facilities;
   (d) the financial circumstances of the patient.
3. The views of the authority on the suitability of the patient for discharge.
4. Any other information or observations on the application which the authority wishes to make.

Responsibility for providing the social circumstances report under point 2 is usually given to the local social services authority and the task undertaken by a mental health social worker, who may or may not be an approved social worker (see Chapter 14).

REFERENCES

Department of Health and Welsh Office (1999). *Mental Health Act 1983: Code of Practice.* London: The Stationery Office.

Gostin, L, Fennell, P (1992). *Mental Health: Tribunal Procedure,* 2nd edn. London: Longman.

10

The Mental Health Act Commission

KEY FACTS

Address and contact details

Mental Health Act Commission
Maid Marian House
56 Hounds Gate
Nottingham NG1 6BG

Tel: 0115 943 7100
Fax: 0115 943 7101
Website: www.mhac.trent.nhs.uk

Chair: Kamlesh Patel
Vice-Chair: Deborah Jenkins
Chief Executive: Chris Heginbotham

Composition

The Mental Health Act Commission was established in 1983. It consists of some 170 members, including lay people, lawyers, doctors, nurses, social workers, psychologists and other specialists. Commissioners are part-time and most are working professionals. They are expected to devote about two days a month to Commission work. The Commission also has a panel of about 150 consultant psychiatrists who operate as second-opinion appointed doctors (SOAD) for the consent to treatment provisions of the Mental Health Act. There is a roughly equal number of men and women on the Commission. The proportion of current Commission members from black and minority ethnic groups is 24 per cent and has increased steadily over the past few years. Commission members fall into two categories: visiting Commission members, whose primary duties include examining statutory documentation, meeting with detained patients, and taking up immediate issues on their behalf, and Commission members, who, in addition, lead the small groups that undertake the visits and write the visit reports.

Functions

The Commission's functions are:

- to keep under review the operation of the Mental Health Act 1983 in respect of patients detained, or liable to be detained under the Act;
- to visit and interview, in private, patients detained under the Act in hospitals and mental nursing homes;
- to investigate complaints that fall within the Commission's remit;
- to appoint medical practitioners and others to give second opinions in cases where this is required by the Act;
- to receive and to examine reports on treatment given under the consent to treatment provisions;
- to submit proposals of forms of medical treatment that should be covered by the safeguards of Section 57 and that give rise to special concern;
- to review decisions to withhold the mail of patients detained in high-security hospitals;
- to publish and lay before Parliament a report every two years;
- to monitor the implementation of the Code of Practice and to propose amendments to ministers;
- to offer advice to ministers on matters falling within the Commission's remit.

The Commission's biennial reports (at the time of writing, the most recent covers the period 2001–03 – Mental Health Act Commission 2003), available from The Stationery Office, are a useful source of material about the operation of the Mental Health Act in England and Wales.

STATUTORY BASIS FOR THE COMMISSION

The Commission is covered by Section 121 of the Mental Health Act 1983. It is a Special Health Authority that carries out functions on behalf of the Secretary of State and the National Assembly for Wales. As the Commission performs functions of a public nature, it is a 'public authority' for the purposes of the Human Rights Act 1998.

It would be possible under the Act for the Secretary of State to extend the Commission's role so that it would cover informal patients, as is the case with the Scottish Mental Welfare Commission. In 1996, the Commission requested that its role should be extended in this way, but the request was denied.

Richard Jones (2002) has criticized the Commission for straying outside its statutory remit (e.g. by examining the physical environment of a hospital). It should also be noted that the Commission has examined guardianship records and has commented on the use of guardianship, although this is outside of its brief. Supervised aftercare would come within the remit of the Commission in so far as a patient will be liable for detention at the point when supervised aftercare arrangements are set up.

THE COMMISSION IN PRACTICE

The Commission has a management board, which is based in Nottingham (at the address given above), together with the administrative staff. For visiting purposes, the Commission is divided into visiting teams (CVTs). There are special teams for high-security hospitals (Broadmoor, Ashworth and Rampton) and seven CVTs that cover England and Wales. These are organized on a regional basis, with about 20 commissioners in each team (e.g. CVT4 covers south-west England).

Most hospitals can expect to be visited three times in a two-year cycle. These visits are usually organized with the hospital concerned in advance, but they can also be on an unannounced basis. Social services departments tend to be visited once every two years, with a particular focus on the work of approved social workers. More information on visits and the general results of past visits can be found in the Commission's biennial reports.

While they are on visits, commissioners usually interview individual patients. The commissioners then leave a letter with the patient to summarize key issues and any action taken. With the patient's permission, a copy is given to the ward manager or a senior member of staff. Statutory records are checked by commissioners, and any action needed is discussed with the hospital concerned. Barnes (1996) has reviewed the Commission's role in protecting detained patients.

In contrast with the Mental Welfare Commission in Scotland, the Mental Health Act Commission does not have any powers to discharge patients. If there are questions over the legality of a patient's detention, then the Commission would need to discuss this with the hospital.

There have been two national visits organized by the Commission where a large number of hospitals were visited on the same day and where there was a focus on a specific issue. The results were then collated and published by the Sainsbury Centre for Mental Health. The second visit, which took place in 2000, focused on detained patients in black and minority ethnic communities (Mental Health Act Commission 2000).

COMPLAINTS

The Commission may be asked to investigate complaints made under Section 120 of the Mental Health Act 1983. Where a complaint concerns the treatment of a patient while he or she was detained, the Commission will usually encourage the person to exhaust the hospital's complaints procedures before taking the matter further.

The Commission also has a policy for dealing with complaints about its own commissioners or SOADs.

The Health Service Ombudsman (2001) has published helpful guidance on complaints in the annual report.

SECOND-OPINION APPOINTED DOCTORS

The Commission appoints a panel of SOADs who visit and give second opinions on certain treatments for patients who are unable or unwilling to give consent under Section 58 of the Mental Health Act. Once appointed, the SOAD exercises his or her independent judgement and decisions cannot be appealed to the Commission. However, decisions could be challenged by way of judicial review. In 2000–01, there were about 6000 requests for SOADs to consider medication and about 2000 requests to consider electroconvulsive therapy (ECT) for patients.

In a Court of Appeal case (*R (on the application of Wooder)* v. *Feggeter and the Mental Health Act Commission* (2002)), it was held that a SOAD owes a duty to give their reasons in writing for requiring a mentally competent patient to be given medication against their will. The SOAD should send a statement of the reasons to the patient's responsible medical officer or to the hospital, and this should be made available for the patient to read. A decision not to disclose could be made only where this would be likely to cause serious harm to the physical or mental health of the patient or of another person.

In 2004 there were 150 SOADs and the Commission recognized in its biennial report that there were difficulties in recruiting working psychiatrists to the panel. One in five SOADs is over retirement age.

INFORMATION

As well as its biennial report, the Mental Health Act Commission publishes patient-information leaflets and practice and guidance notes. These include guidance on statutory forms and matters such as the use of medication. The Commission also drew attention to the problems of deaths of patients (sometimes attributed to prescribed medication) in a climate where risks posed by patients were getting more attention (Mental Health Act Commission 2001).

FUTURE OF THE MENTAL HEALTH ACT COMMISSION

This is rather uncertain at the time of writing. The Draft Mental Health Bill (Department of Health 2002) made no specific mention of the Commission, and it was expected that the Mental Health Act Commission would be subsumed within the Commission for Health Improvement. However, there have been arguments that it should retain a separate identity within any reformed Commission for Health Improvement. As the Mental Health Bill was omitted from the Queen's Speech in November 2002, the position is somewhat unclear, but the Commission is likely to continue in its present form for the next couple of years at least.

REFERENCES

Barnes, M (1996). Citizens in detention: the role of the Mental Health Act Commission in protecting the rights of detained patients. *Local Government Studies* **22**, 28–46.

Department of Health (2002). *Draft Mental Health Bill Cmnd 5538*. London: The Stationery Office.

Health Service Ombudsman (2001). *Health Service Ombudsman's Annual Report 2000–01*. London: The Stationery Office.

Jones, R (2002). *Mental Health Act Manual*, 8th edn. London: Sweet and Maxwell.

Mental Health Act Commission (2000). *National Visit 2: Improving Care for Detained Patients in Black and Minority Ethnic Communities*. London: Sainsbury Centre for Mental Health.

Mental Health Act Commission (2001). *Deaths of Detained Patients in England and Wales: a Report by the Mental Health Act Commission on Information Collected from 1 February 1997 to January 2000*. Nottingham: Mental Health Act Commission.

Mental Health Act Commission (2003) *Placed Amongst Strangers: Tenth Biennial Report*. London: The Stationery Office.

11

The Code of Practice, including its legal standing

THIRD EDITION OF THE CODE OF PRACTICE

The revised Code of Practice to the Mental Health Act 1983 came into force in 1999. This replaced the second edition, which had been in place since November 1993. The Mental Health Act Commission suggested changes to the Secretary of State for Health, and a revised Code was expected in 1997. However, a number of factors contributed to a delay, and the Code was finally laid before Parliament in December 1998. The main reasons for the delay were a change in the government; some high-profile cases where hospital managers had discharged detained patients against clinical advice; and several cases that affected the law on admission, detention and treatment. These cases are referred to in more detail elsewhere and include the Bournewood Trust case (*R* v. *Bournewood Community and Mental Health NHS Trust ex parte L* (1998) All ER 319), on informal admission, and *R* v. *Collins* (*R* v. *Collins and others ex parte S* (1998) COD 396), which considered the grounds for detention as well as some specific treatment issues. Mental incapacity was a central concern in these cases.

Guiding principles are brought together in Chapter 1 of the Code and should be read as background to the other chapters. The revised version of the memorandum (Department of Health 1998) was published in 1998. It is frequently referenced and needs to be read alongside the Code.

PURPOSE OF THE CODE OF PRACTICE

Paragraph 2 of the introduction to the Code states:

> The Code provides guidance to registered medical practitioners, managers and staff of hospitals and mental nursing homes, and approved social workers (ASWs) (who have defined responsibilities under the provisions of the Act), on how to proceed when undertaking duties under the Act. It should also be considered by others working in health and social services (including the independent and voluntary sectors), and by the police.

The introduction expresses the hope that the Code will be a help to patients, their families, their friends and others who support them and notes that it was drafted with this aim in mind. Certainly many will find the language more accessible than the Act or the Regulations (Department of Health (1983) Mental Health (hospital, guardianship and consent to treatment) Regulations 1983, SI 1983, no. 893).

STATUS OF THE CODE OF PRACTICE IN LEGAL AND OTHER PROCEEDINGS

The Code was prepared in accordance with Section 118 of the Act. The introduction to the Code notes in the first paragraph that the Act 'does not impose a legal duty to comply with the Code but as it is a statutory document, failure to follow it could be referred to in evidence in legal proceedings'. The effect of non-compliance with the Code would depend on the circumstances. In the recent Court of Appeal case of *R (on the application of Munjaz)* v. *Mersey Care NHS Trust* (2003)), the Court held that the Code must be followed unless there are good reasons for departing from it in relation to a particular patient. This judgment has, in effect, raised the status of the Code of Practice, and those working to the Act should ensure that they are familiar with the Code's guidance.

The Code might be relevant in the case of a potential action against a member of staff. Section 139 of the Mental Health Act provides some safeguards for staff against vexatious actions from patients. The patient would need to establish in the High Court that the member of staff had acted in bad faith or without reasonable care and a breach of the Code might be used in this context. Interestingly, Hoggett (1996, p. 250) argues against the need for Section 139 and considers that 'patients are in a peculiarly powerless position which merits, if anything, extra safeguards rather than the removal of those available to everyone else'.

The Code may also be referred to in inquiries and in disciplinary proceedings, and it behoves those operating under the Mental Health Act to at least give consideration to the Code's guidance. In some situations, they may be unable to follow it because of lack of resources or possibly having received their own legal advice that they should not do so for some specific reason (e.g. recent case law).

POLICY REQUIREMENTS IN THE CODE OF PRACTICE

The Code contains a number of policy requirements. Most of these are directed at health or local authorities. For example, Paragraph 2.38 requires local authorities to have explicit policies on how to respond to repeated requests from nearest relatives for an assessment under Section 13(4) of the Act. This recognizes the potential stress as well as the resource implications of carrying out repeated assessments when nothing has changed. Chapter 21 includes a requirement for the hospital managers to have a policy covering what action should be taken if a detained patient goes absent without leave.

GUIDING PRINCIPLES

Guiding principles are gathered together at the beginning of the Code, and this first chapter needs to be read before considering any of the specific advice in the other chapters. The principles include (at Paragraph 1.1) statements that people to whom the Act applies should:

> … receive recognition for their basic human rights under the European Convention of Human Rights … be given respect for their qualities, abilities and diverse backgrounds as individuals and be assured that account will be taken of their age, gender, sexual orientation, social, cultural and religious background, but that general assumptions will not be made on the basis of any one of these characteristics … be given any necessary treatment or care in the least controlled and segregated facilities compatible with ensuring their own health or safety or the safety of other people; be discharged from detention or other powers provided by the Act as soon as it is clear that their application is no longer justified.

COMMUNICATING WITH PATIENTS AND THE USE OF INTERPRETERS

The Code advises that staff should ensure that effective communication takes place between themselves and their patients. It stresses that information may need to be given on a number of different occasions. Paragraph 1.11 might be seen as providing some compensation for a lack of protection in this area for patients in guardianship and for mentally incapacitated patients who are admitted informally to hospital. Because of its significance it is reprinted here in full:

> All patients, including those subject to guardianship, should be given full information, both verbally and in writing to help them understand why they are in hospital, or subject to guardianship, and the care and treatment they will be given. Informal patients who are capable of expressing consent should be told they may leave at any time. Where mentally incapacitated patients have been admitted informally their position should be explained to them as far as possible and their close relative, carer or advocate should be kept informed about the arrangements for their care.

The issue of mental incapacity will be considered in more detail below when looking at changes in the definition of an informal inpatient.

The Code places an increased emphasis on good practice in the use of interpreters. It states at Paragraph 1.4:

> … Local and Health Authorities and Trusts should ensure that ASWs, doctors, nurses and others receive sufficient guidance in the use of interpreters, and should make arrangements for there to be an easily accessible pool of trained interpreters. Authorities and Trusts should consider co-operating in making this provision.

In terms of practice, the Code indicates that patients' relatives or friends should not normally be used as an intermediary or interpreter. The Code considers situations where the patient's first language is not English, there are hearing or visual impairments, or there are other barriers to communication.

CONFIDENTIALITY

The Code stresses that in normal circumstances, information about a patient should be disclosed only with the patient's consent, but it recognizes that occasionally it may be necessary to pass on particular information to professionals or others in the public interest, e.g. where personal health or safety is at risk.

There is some specific advice about the position of patients detained under Part III of the Act (which applies to those who were concerned in criminal proceedings or under sentence).

INFORMAL ADMISSION

The definition of an informal patient was central to the Bournewood case. The various references to informal patients in the Code reflect the law lords' judgment. As the Bournewood case is now to be heard in the European Court in Strasbourg, what follows will need to be revised in the light of whatever judgment that court reaches in due course. The Code considers matters based on the law lords' view. For example, Paragraph 2.8 states:

> If at the time of admission, the patient is mentally incapable of consent, but does not object to entering hospital and receiving care or treatment, admission should be informal … The decision to admit a mentally incapacitated patient informally should be made by the doctor in charge of the patient's treatment in accordance with what is in the patient's best interests and is justifiable on the basis of the common law doctrine of necessity … If a patient lacks capacity at the time of an assessment or review, it is particularly important that both clinical and social care requirements are considered, and that account is taken of the patient's ascertainable wishes and feelings and the views of their immediate relatives and carers on what would be in the patient's best interests.

In Chapter 30 of the Code, which considers people with learning disabilities, Paragraph 30.6 makes a similar statement:

> A person who has severe learning disabilities and lacks the capacity to make personal health care decisions may be admitted to hospital on an informal basis if he or she does not object to being an in-patient. In that case the patient's admission and care must be in his or her best interests and in accordance with the common law doctrine of necessity.

The 1993 Code had a rather contentious definition of what would constitute an informal inpatient in relation to the doctor's holding power under Section 5(2). Essentially, it described an informal patient as:

... one who has understood and accepted an offer of a bed, who has freely appeared on the ward and who has co-operated with the admission procedure.

Jones (1996, p. 586) noted:

> ... only patients who are both mentally competent and willing to co-operate with the admission process would come within the scope of this definition. As the wording of the Act does not support an approach which would have the effect of excluding patients who do not possess such characteristics from the application of the holding power, a better definition would be: 'An informal patient for the purpose of this section, is one who has arrived on the ward and who has offered no resistance to the admission procedure'.

This view was specifically contradicted in October 1997 at the Appeal Court stage of the Bournewood case, but it was, in effect, then supported by the law lords' ruling in June 1998. The eight-month period in between led to some interesting responses. It is instructive to compare Jones' suggestion with the equivalent paragraph in the revised Code, which now reads:

> 8.4 For the purposes of section 5(2) informal patients are usually voluntary patients, i.e. those who have the capacity to consent and who consent to enter hospital for inpatient treatment. Patients who lack the capacity to consent but do not object to admission for treatment may also be informal patients ... The section cannot be used for an outpatient attending a hospital's accident and emergency department. Admission procedures should not be implemented with the sole intention of then using the power in section 5(2).

There is no requirement in the Code that Trusts have clear written statements on what constitutes the admission procedure, but many will find it helpful to do so.

The whole area of mental incapacity is contentious in light of the current review of the Mental Health Act. The government has now introduced a Mental Capacity Bill to Parliament. This will overlap significantly with the Mental Health Act in that it will provide for certain decisions (including admission to hospital and consent to treatment) to be taken on someone else's behalf. In the meantime, the Code provides some more recent guidance than has previously been available to staff.

MENTAL CAPACITY AND MEDICAL TREATMENT

Chapter 15 of the Code covers general issues concerning medical treatment. It notes that, under common law, valid consent is required before medical treatment can be given, except where common law or statute provides authority to give treatment without consent. However, the basic principles of consent are reworded to reflect more recent views. Paragraph 15.13 notes:

'Consent' is the voluntary and continuing permission of the patient to receive a particular treatment, based on an adequate knowledge of the purpose, nature, likely effects and risks of that treatment including the likelihood of its success and any alternatives to it. Permission given under any unfair or undue pressure is not 'consent'.

The assessment of a patient's capacity to make a decision about their own medical treatment is a matter for clinical judgment.

Basic principles on capacity have been reworded to reflect recent cases (*Re C (refusal of Treatment)* (1994) 1 FLR 31, *Re MB* (1997) 2 FCR 541). According to Paragraph 15.10 of the Code, an individual is presumed to have capacity to make a treatment decision unless he or she:

- is unable to take in and retain the information material to the decision especially as to the likely consequences of having or not having the treatment; or
- is unable to believe the information; or
- is unable to weigh the information in the balance as part of a process of arriving at the decision.

There is recognition that any assessment must relate to the particular treatment or admission proposal and that capacity may vary over time. Any assessment of a person's capacity should be recorded in the patient's medical notes.

Paragraph 15.11 of the Code addresses the issue of advance directives and states that to be valid:

… an advance refusal must be clearly verifiable and must relate to the type of treatment now proposed. If there is any reason to doubt the reliability of an advance refusal of treatment, then an application to the court for a declaration could be made. The individual must have had the capacity to make an advance refusal when it was made. An advanced refusal of medical treatment for mental disorder does not prevent the authorization of such treatment by Part IV of the Act in the circumstances where those provisions apply.

In relation to advance directives, the Code also refers to the guidelines that are set out in the judgment *R* v. *Collins ex parte S (no. 2)* (in particular, guideline no. 3 in *R* v. *Collins ex parte S (no. 2)* (1998)).

The Code contains more detailed guidance on treatment of people without capacity to consent. It notes that an adult may be mentally incapable of consenting to, or refusing, treatment as a result of temporary factors such as delirium, shock, pain or drugs; in some cases, this may be more long-lasting, as with patients with severe learning disabilities and some patients with Alzheimer's disease.

Again referring to the Bournewood case and in looking at those who lack capacity to consent, the Code comments that there are considerations that doctors must have in discharging their duty of care: 'Treatment for their condition may be prescribed … in their best interests under the common law doctrine of necessity.'

In the same paragraph (15.21) in referring to the case of *Re F* (*Re F* (1990) 2 AC 1), the Code states: 'if treatment is given to a patient who is not capable of giving consent "in the patient's best interests"', then the treatment must be:

... necessary to save life or prevent a deterioration or ensure an improvement in the patient's physical or mental health; and in accordance with a practice accepted at the time by a reasonable body of medical opinion skilled in the particular form of treatment in question.

In exceptional circumstances, a proposed treatment should not be carried out without first seeking the approval of the High Court by way of a declaration. The rules of Part IV of the Act do not apply to the treatment of physical disorders unless it can be said reasonably that the physical disorder is a symptom or underlying cause of the mental disorder (*B* v. *Croydon Health Authority* (1995) 2 WLR 294). The Code states that, if in doubt, the responsible medical officer should seek legal advice.

CHILDREN AND MEDICAL TREATMENT

The chapter on children and young people was revised significantly in the 1999 version of the Code. A major part of the chapter links with the issues of capacity and valid consent, which we have just considered. The implications of the Gillick case (*Gillick* v. *West Norfolk and Wisbech Area Health Authority* (1986) AC112) and subsequent rulings are considered. The Code states at Paragraph 31.11:

A 'Gillick competent' child can give a valid consent to medical treatment. A child may be regarded as 'Gillick competent' if the doctor concludes that he or she has the capacity to make the decision to have the proposed treatment and is of sufficient understanding and intelligence to be capable of making up his/her own mind.

The Code recognizes, however, that, as with the case of a young person with anorexia nervosa, the refusal of a 'Gillick competent' child to be treated medically can be overridden by the courts or by the child's parents (*Re W* (1992) All ER 627).

Paragraph 31.13 clarifies circumstances where court assistance may be sought:

in the case of a child who is not 16 or Gillick competent where treatment decisions need to be made and the person with parental responsibility cannot be identified or is incapacitated, e.g. in dealing with a child who is accommodated by a local authority;
where a person with parental responsibility may not be acting in the best interests of the child in making treatment decisions on behalf of the child.

A child's refusal to be treated is a very important consideration in making clinical judgements and for parents and the court in deciding whether themselves to give consent. Its importance increases with age and maturity of the child.

The Code notes that where children are subjects of emergency protection orders, child assessment orders, interim care orders or full supervision orders, the Children Act specifically provides that they may refuse assessment, examination or treatment but also that the inherent jurisdiction of the High Court can be used to override a child's refusal, where it considers it should do so.

SUPERVISED AFTERCARE

Aftercare under supervision (also sometimes known as supervised discharge) is summarized in Chapter 28 of the Code. However, there is also a supplement to the Code that covers supervised aftercare (in England, see HSG(96)11/ LAC(96)8 *Guidance on Supervised Discharge and Related Provisions*; in Wales, see WHC(96)11 *Guidance on Supervised Discharge and Related Provisions*).

CONCLUSION: A LOOK TO THE FUTURE

The Code's advice and guidance on issues relating to mental incapacity have proved to be the most controversial and, to some extent, the most difficult to follow. To a large degree, this reflects the unsatisfactory position where much of the relevant law is not yet in statute but where practitioners are expecting it to be in the future. There is a view that a comprehensive act covering mental incapacity might remove the need for any separate act on mental disorder. At the time of writing, it seems unlikely that the final version of the expected Mental Capacity Act will be so comprehensive as to replace the Mental Health Act, but it will have a significant impact on its operation.

Current concerns in the areas of personality disorder and of risks to the public, to patients and to their carers, may also influence the three strands of the present review of legislation: mental incapacity, the Mental Health Act, and personality disorder. It will be instructive to look at parallel developments in Northern Ireland, Scotland and other parts of Europe, and one may perhaps hope for some clearer, more integrated approach to the law than has been the recent experience. Within this context, the revised Code provided a small step forward in addressing some of the key issues. However, its effectiveness in protecting the rights and quality of service for those affected by the Act depends largely on the responses of staff and of those who provide the resources, support and guidance that are necessary.

REFERENCES

Department of Health (1998). *Mental Health Act 1983: Memorandum on Parts I to VI, VIII and X.* London: HMSO.

Hoggett, B (1996). *Mental Health Law*, 4th edn. London: Sweet and Maxwell.

Jones, R (1996). *Mental Health Act Manual*, 5th edn. London: Sweet & Maxwell.

12

Removal and return of patients to and from England and Wales

The Mental Health Act 1983 applies to England and Wales, while other parts of the UK (Scotland, Northern Ireland, the Channel Islands and the Isle of Man) have their own mental health legislation. Occasionally, psychiatric patients who are currently detained in hospital or are under guardianship may need to be removed or returned within the UK. Part VI of the Mental Health Act 1983 provides the necessary legislation to allow the transfer of such patients across national boundaries within the UK without any break in the power for confinement. Similarly, provision is also made (under Section 86 of Part VI of the Act) for the removal of psychiatric patients who are aliens.

REMOVAL TO SCOTLAND

Section 80 of the Mental Health Act 1983 allows for the transfer of psychiatric patients who are currently detained in hospital or are under guardianship from England or Wales to Scotland without any break in the power for confinement.

Unrestricted patients

Section 80(1) of the Mental Health Act 1983 applies to the case of patients in England and Wales who are either liable to detention without restriction on discharge (apart from patients remanded for report or treatment or subject to an interim hospital order, i.e. excluding sections 35, 36 and 38, respectively) or subject to guardianship under the Act. If it appears to the Secretary of State that it is in the interests of such a patient that he or she be removed to Scotland, and that arrangements have been made for either admitting the patient to a hospital or receiving the patient into guardianship, as required, then, under Section 80 of the Mental Health Act 1983, the Secretary of State may authorize the patient's removal to Scotland and may give any necessary directions for his or her conveyance to their destination. Such a patient is to be treated in Scotland as if subject to the corresponding section of the Mental Health (Scotland) Act (see Chapter 21).

Section 80(4) of the Mental Health Act 1983 applies to the case of a patient removed to Scotland from England or Wales such that the patient was liable, immediately before removal, to be detained under an order for admission to hospital for assessment under the Mental Health Act 1983. On admission to a hospital in Scotland, the patient is to be treated as if he or she had been admitted subject to an emergency recommendation under the Mental Health (Scotland) Act (see Chapter 21), made on the date of his or her admission.

Section 80(5) of the Mental Health Act 1983 applies to the case of a patient removed to Scotland from England or Wales such that the patient was subject, immediately before removal, to a transfer direction given while he or she was serving a sentence of imprisonment (under Section 47 of the Act) imposed by a court in England or Wales. Such a patient is to be treated as if the sentence had been imposed by a court in Scotland.

Restricted patients

Section 80(6) of the Mental Health Act 1983 applies to the case of a patient removed to Scotland from England or Wales such that the patient was subject, immediately before removal, to a restriction order or restriction direction of limited duration. The date of expiry of the restriction order or restriction direction is not changed by the removal to Scotland.

REMOVAL TO ENGLAND OR WALES

Reciprocal arrangements exist between England and Wales and Scotland with respect to psychiatric patients removed from Scotland to England or Wales.

REMOVAL TO AND FROM NORTHERN IRELAND

Sections 81 and 82 of the Mental Health Act 1983 allow for the transfer of psychiatric patients who are currently detained in hospital or are under guardianship between England or Wales and Northern Ireland without any break in the power for confinement.

Unrestricted patients

Section 81(1) of the Mental Health Act 1983 applies to the case of patients in England and Wales who are either liable to detention without restriction on discharge (apart from patients remanded for report or treatment or subject to an interim hospital order, i.e. excluding sections 35, 36 and 38, respectively) or subject to guardianship under the Act. If it appears to the Secretary of State that it is in the interests of such a patient that he or she be removed to Northern Ireland, and that arrangements have been made for either admitting the patient

to a hospital or receiving the patient into guardianship, as required, then, under Section 81 of the Mental Health Act 1983, the Secretary of State may authorize the patient's removal to Northern Ireland and may give any necessary directions for his or her conveyance to their destination. Such a patient is to be treated in Northern Ireland as if subject to the corresponding enactment of the Mental Health (Northern Ireland) Order (see Chapter 21).

Section 81(4) of the Mental Health Act 1983 applies to the case of a patient removed to Northern Ireland from England or Wales such that the patient was liable, immediately before removal, to be detained under an order for admission to hospital for assessment under the Mental Health Act 1983. On admission to a hospital in Northern Ireland, the patient is to be treated as if he or she had been admitted in pursuance of an application for assessment under Article 4 of the Mental Health (Northern Ireland) Order 1986 (see Chapter 21), made on the date of his or her admission.

Section 81(5) of the Mental Health Act 1983 applies to the case of a patient removed to Northern Ireland from England or Wales such that the patient was liable, immediately before removal, to be detained under an order for admission to hospital for treatment under the Mental Health Act 1983. On admission to a hospital in Northern Ireland, the patient is to be treated as if he or she had been admitted subject to detention for treatment under Part II of the Mental Health (Northern Ireland) Order 1986 (see Chapter 21), made on the date of his or her admission.

Section 81(6) of the Mental Health Act 1983 applies to the case of a patient removed to Northern Ireland from England or Wales such that the patient was subject, immediately before removal, to a transfer direction given while he or she was serving a sentence of imprisonment (under Section 47 of the Act) imposed by a court in England or Wales. Such a patient is to be treated as if the sentence had been imposed by a court in Northern Ireland.

Restricted patients

Section 81(7) of the Mental Health Act 1983 applies to the case of a patient removed to Northern Ireland from England or Wales such that the patient was subject, immediately before removal, to a restriction order or restriction direction of limited duration. The date of expiry of the restriction order or restriction direction is not changed by the removal to Northern Ireland.

Removal to England or Wales

Reciprocal arrangements exist between England and Wales and Northern Ireland with respect to psychiatric patients removed from Northern Ireland to England or Wales. These are covered by Section 82 of the Mental Health Act 1983.

REMOVAL TO AND FROM THE CHANNEL ISLANDS AND THE ISLE OF MAN

Sections 83 and 85 of the Mental Health Act 1983 allow for the transfer of psychiatric patients who are currently detained in hospital or are under guardianship between England or Wales and the Channel Islands or the Isle of Man without any break in the power for confinement. Section 84 of the Mental Health Act 1983 allows for the removal from the Channel Islands or the Isle of Man to England or Wales of an offender found to be insane.

Removal to the Channel Islands or the Isle of Man

Section 83 of the Mental Health Act 1983 applies to the case of patients in England and Wales who are either liable to detention without restriction on discharge (apart from patients remanded for report or treatment or subject to an interim hospital order, i.e. excluding sections 35, 36 and 38, respectively) or subject to guardianship under the Act. If it appears to the Secretary of State that it is in the interests of such a patient that he or she be removed to the Channel Islands or the Isle of Man, and that arrangements have been made for either admitting the patient to a hospital or receiving the patient into guardianship, as required, then, under Section 83 of the Mental Health Act 1983, the Secretary of State may authorize the patient's removal to the Channel Islands or the Isle of Man and may give any necessary directions for his or her conveyance to their destination.

Removal of offenders found to be insane from the Channel Islands or the Isle of Man

Section 84 of the Mental Health Act 1983 allows for the transfer of offenders found to be insane from the Channel Islands or the Isle of Man, where the necessary hospital facilities are not available, to such facilities in England and Wales.

The Secretary of State (which, in this case, is the Home Secretary) may by warrant direct that any offender found by a court in any of the Channel Islands or in the Isle of Man to be insane or to have been insane at the time of the alleged offence, and ordered to be detained during Her Majesty's pleasure, be removed to a hospital in England and Wales. Such a patient, on reception into the hospital in England or Wales, is treated as if he or she had been removed to that hospital under Section 46 of the Mental Health Act 1983. Also, the Home Secretary may direct that any such removed patient be returned to the island from which he or she was removed to be dealt with there according to law in all respects as if the patient had not been removed under this section.

Removal to England or Wales

Reciprocal arrangements exist between, on the one hand, England and Wales and, on the other hand, the Channel Islands and the Isle of Man, with respect to psychiatric patients removed from the Channel Islands or the Isle of Man to England or Wales. These are covered by Section 85 of the Mental Health Act 1983.

In the case of such a patient who is subject to an order or direction restricting his or her discharge, the patient is treated as if subject to a restriction order or restriction direction. While being conveyed to the hospital in England or Wales, such a patient is deemed to be in legal custody. (Under these circumstances, Section 138 applies to the patient as if he or she were in legal custody by virtue of Section 137.)

REMOVAL OF ALIENS

Section 86 of the Mental Health Act 1983 applies to any patient who is:

- not a British citizen;
- not a Commonwealth citizen having the right of abode in the UK by virtue of Section 2(1)(b) of the Immigration Act 1971;
- receiving treatment for mental illness as an inpatient in a hospital in England or Wales under certain provisions of the Mental Health Act 1983 (other than under sections 35, 36 or 38) or in Northern Ireland under the Mental Health (Northern Ireland) Order 1986.

Section 86 does not apply to informal patients or to those granted extended leave of absence under Section 17.

If it appears to the Secretary of State (the Home Secretary) that proper arrangements (including travel arrangements and nurse escorts) have been made for the removal of such a patient to a country or territory outside the UK, the Isle of Man or the Channel Islands and for his or her care or treatment there, and that it is in the interests of the patient to remove him or her, then, only with the approval of a Mental Health Review Tribunal (or, in the case of Northern Ireland, the Mental Health Review Tribunal for Northern Ireland), the Secretary of State may:

- by warrant authorize the removal of the patient from the place where he or she is receiving treatment;
- give directions for the conveyance of the patient to his or her destination in that country or territory and for his or her detention in any place or on board any ship or aircraft until his or her arrival at any specified port or place in any such country or territory.

If a restriction order is in force, then it continues to apply should the patient return to England or Wales before the date on which the restriction order would have expired if the patient had remained in England or Wales.

Application to the Home Office is usually not required in the case of patients who are willing to travel and for whom suitable arrangements have been made.

In their experience, Green and Nayani (2000) have found that the following steps are required in order to arrange repatriation:

- Contact the relevant embassy.
- Arrange for an interpreter in order to interview the patient (and his or her relatives), if necessary.
- Obtain information regarding previous contact with psychiatric services in the patient's country of origin and establish which hospital in that country should be responsible for the patient's care.

- Obtain specific information regarding the patient's past psychiatric history, including previous diagnosis, treatment, response to treatment and any history of dangerousness.
- Translation of correspondence.
- Continue treatment until the patient is fit to travel.
- Consider repatriation (under Section 86, if necessary) and discuss this with the patient.
- Arrange the date and process of transfer.

Green and Nayani (2000) suggest the following useful questions to ask embassy staff:

- Have you been involved in repatriating psychiatric patients?
- Will you find information about which hospital the patient should return to?
- Will you liaise directly with the hospital concerned to obtain information regarding the patient's past psychiatric history and to arrange plans for transfer?
- Will you be able to translate discharge summaries and other correspondence, and will there be a charge for this?
- If the patient is detained in this country under the Mental Health Act, is there any process ensuring the patient remains detained from the time they leave England [or Wales] until the time they arrive in the appropriate hospital?
- Does the patient return directly to his/her local hospital or is he [or she] assessed at a central hospital initially?
- Who is responsible for the cost of repatriation?

REFERENCE

Green, L, Nayani, T (2000). Repatriating psychiatric patients. *Psychiatric Bulletin* **24**, 405–8.

13

Management of property and affairs of patients

INTRODUCTION

Most people are capable of managing their own affairs. They have a working life, they may own their own home and have other property and a bank account, and they do not require additional help.

Issues relating to other people managing property and affairs are primarily of importance to the elderly, but they can also apply to younger people with mental health problems such as mania and who have substantial assets.

In the mental health field, particularly in elderly people, it is important to consider people's capacity to manage affairs and to protect them from financial abuse.

ENDURING POWER OF ATTORNEY

Enduring Power of Attorney (EPA) is a legal device enabling someone else, an attorney, to manage a person's affairs, usually when the person has become incapable or has found the management of their affairs too onerous. Usually the person is elderly and a member of the family seeks assistance on their behalf.

An ordinary Power of Attorney is simply a deed executed by a person, the donor, who appoints someone, the attorney, to act on his or her behalf. This can be for a limited purpose and time, such as the sale of a house while the owner is abroad. The deed can also give a general power but is revoked automatically and ceases to be valid when the donor becomes incapable.

The **Enduring Power of Attorney Act 1985** was introduced to provide for people who later become incapable through mental disorder. It can remain in force when they are incapable provided it is registered with the Public Trust Office. EPA is designed to be a cheaper, less restrictive and more individual form of managing affairs than the Court of Protection.

There is some loss of security because of this, and there are occasions when financial abuse occurs. However, there are very many EPAs in force, and the majority of them enable a person's affairs to be managed cheaply and competently by someone of their choice without any problems.

The EPA is drawn up on a special form, which is available from a law stationer's office. It is recommended that a solicitor draws up the EPA. It must be completed by, or on behalf of, the person giving the power, and it must be signed in the presence of a witness. The attorney must also sign to show that he or she agrees to act on behalf of the person and that he or she understands the duty to register when and if the donor becomes incapable.

An EPA may have more than one attorney, who may act jointly or severally. Joint appointments mean that all attorneys must act together over any action, which gives greater security to the donor. It is less convenient, as all attorneys have to meet, and it also increases the risk of failure because of death or incapacity.

Joint and several appointments mean that any one of the attorneys may act alone. The EPA may be limited to one aspect of the donor's affairs or may be general. It can also be a general power with restrictions. General powers apply only to financial affairs, and not to health or social affairs. The donor may choose to have the EPA take effect immediately or to have it postponed until he or she becomes incapable. The attorney cannot take any action that would benefit him- or herself or anyone else other than the donor, but the attorney can make gifts such as Christmas, wedding and birthday presents; the most common form of abuse of an EPA lies in excessive gifting.

REGISTRATION

Registration should be done as soon as possible after the donor becomes incapable. Official notification should be sent to all attorneys as well as the donor and three relatives who are designated in order of importance. No medical evidence is required to verify the donor's incapacity.

When the attorney applies for registration, the EPA is suspended until it is complete. After the EPA is registered successfully, it becomes irrevocable, except with the consent of the Court of Protection. The donor and relatives have an opportunity to object to the attorneys and to registration at the time of registration.

The Act does not specify the degree of mental capacity required for the creation of the EPA. It does define the mental incapacity needed for registration to help the attorney to know when to register the EPA. This should occur when the attorney has reason to believe that the donor is 'incapable, by reason of mental disorder, of managing and administering his own property and affairs'.

The capacity required to execute an EPA was considered in the case of *Re K, Re F* (1988) ALL ER 1988 Vol. 1. In this case, an elderly woman signed an EPA and an application to register was submitted a short time later. She was asked whether she had been capable of understanding what an EPA was when she signed the initial application. It was accepted that at the time she created the EPA, she understood its nature and effect but was not capable of managing her affairs.

The question then arose as to whether the EPA was valid. Hoffman J held that the test was whether the donor had the capacity to understand the nature and power of the EPA. He set out four aspects that a person must understand in order to be able to give assent:

- that the attorney will be able to assume complete authority over the donor's affairs;

- that the attorney will be able to do anything with the property that the donor would have done;
- that the authority will continue if the donor becomes incapable;
- that when the donor becomes incapable, the power will become irrevocable without the consent of the Court of Protection.

It was recommended that the donor should not have the power explained and then be asked 'Do you understand?' in such a way that the answer can only be 'Yes' or 'No'. Instead, the donor should be asked to explain in his or her own words what the attorney can do, which is a more meaningful assessment of the donor's understanding of the powers of an EPA. This safeguards people who do not understand but have appropriate social skills and know when to agree with people.

COURT OF PROTECTION

The Court of Protection is an office of the Supreme Court in England and Wales that is required to protect and manage the property and affairs of mentally disordered people who are incapable of managing their own affairs.

Recently, there have been many more applications because of the property boom. Mrs Macfarlane, former Master of the Court of Protection, in 1987 reported that 82 per cent of the court cases were over the age of 55 years and the majority were women suffering from senile dementia. The staffing in the Public Trust Office has not increased correspondingly.

The powers of the Court of Protection are derived from Part VII of the Mental Health Act 1983 and supplemented by the Court of Protection Rules 1994.

The Court can deal only with financial, legal, business and property transactions. It has no power over any form of medical treatment; nor can it dictate about a person's social circumstances.

Communication with the Court is almost exclusively by correspondence and telephone. In practice, applications are made to the court by solicitors, local authorities, social service departments and relatives. This can be done by a written application (Form CPI) accompanied by a completed certificate about the property of the patient (Form GP5) and a medical certificate (Form CP3), together with the appropriate fee.

Medical certificate

Only one medical certificate is required to show the existence of a mental disorder and incapacity. This can be by either the patient's general practitioner (GP) or a consultant psychiatrist. There is concern that only one opinion need be supplied and that the form should contain sufficient information so that the court can judge. The information need not include a diagnosis but in practice there will be problems if one only describes the symptoms of schizophrenia without naming the disorder.

Receivership

The Court operates by appointing someone to manage the patient's affairs on their behalf who is called a receiver. The most suitable receivers are relatives or friends; statistics for 1991 show that two-thirds of receivers are relatives. The Court will require a reference and guarantee bond as a safeguard, but solicitors, accountants and bank managers can also take receivership for a fee paid by the patient to safeguard their assets. If no suitable receiver can be found, then the Court appoints the Public Trustee. Receiverships are monitored by the Court through the Receiverships Division of the Public Trust Office, and the Court should be contacted immediately if it is thought that a receiver is abusing his or her powers. A receiver must keep proper accounts and act for the patient in financial matters. Selling a house will require further specific authorization from the Court. This affords the patient more protection than does the EPA.

The whole system is slow, bureaucratic, understaffed and geographically remote, and it can be very expensive.

APPOINTEESHIP

In smaller cases in which it is not possible to use the Court of Protection because there is little money involved, but the person has not made any advance preparation and is incapable of managing his or her affairs, an appointeeship can be set up. This is a statutory procedure carried out under Regulation 33 of the **Social Security (Claims and Payments) Regulations 1987**. The appointee has to apply to the Benefits Agency, which will make suitable enquiries and interview the appointee. The appointee is usually a professional, such as a social worker, who is appointed officially, but it can also be a relative. The appointee will then have the person's benefits book printed in their name indefinitely. This practical measure is done infrequently (about one per cent of all benefits claims) due to rules and regulations prohibiting professionals taking it up.

WILLS

In England and Wales, the execution of wills is governed by the **Wills Act (1837, 1861, 1863 and 1968)** and, in some circumstances, the Mental Health Act 1983. These statutes are augmented by a large amount of case law.

Under the **Administration of Estates Act 1925**, the Intestacy Rules apply when a person dies without making a will. A surviving spouse, if there is one, will get the deceased person's personal effects and a legacy of £125 000 if there are children or £200 000 if there are no children and a share in the rest of the estate, depending on which relatives survive.

The Crown will take the entire estate if there is nobody on the list.

MENTAL CAPACITY

In the index case of *Banks* v. *Goodfellow* (1870) LR 5 QP 549, Cockburn CJ said eloquently:

> It is essential ... that a testator shall understand the nature of the act and its effects, shall understand the extent of the property of which he is disposing, shall be able to comprehend and appreciate the claims to which he ought to give effect, and with a view to the latter object, that no disorder and mind shall poison his affections, pervert his sense of right, or prevent the exercise of his natural faculties – that no insane delusion shall influence his will in disposing of his property and bring about a disposal of it which, if the mind has been sound, would not have been made. Any person making a Will must intend to make it the way it is set out so that it reflects his real wishes.

Vulnerable elderly people may easily be pressured into making a will in favour of a particular person and 'undue influence' is described in the case of *Hall* v. *Hall* (1968) as coercion to overpower the volition but without convincing the judgement.

When making a will, the testator must have the intention to make that particular will.

CONCLUSIONS

In this chapter, we have seen a range of provisions for people who are unable to manage their financial affairs due to mental disorder:

- the EPA, which is simple and cheap to run but can be open to abuse;
- the Court of Protection, which is a more formalized procedure with a lot more safeguards but is costly and slow;
- the Appointeeship, which is a practical measure for people on state benefits and who cannot manage their affairs, but this is probably underused;
- finally, most people are able to make wills, but for those who cannot it is sometimes possible for a will to be made under the Court of Protection.

14

Approved social workers

INTRODUCTION

The significance of the role of the approved social worker (ASW) in current law was underlined by Lord Bingham in part of the judgment on a recent House of Lords case (*R* v. *East London & the City Mental Health NHS Trust and another (Respondents) ex parte von Brandenburg (aka Hanley)* (2003)). In this case, an ASW had applied for a patient's detention under Section 3 where a Mental Health Review Tribunal had, six days earlier, ordered the patient's discharge from Section 2. The discharge was due to take effect the day after the Section 3 application. In ruling on the circumstances in which such an application would be illegal, Lord Bingham stated:

> I would, secondly, resist the lumping together of the ASW and the recommending doctor or doctors as 'the mental health professionals'. It is the ASW who makes the application, not the doctors.

The ASW was seen as carrying the primary responsibility for not flying in the face of a Tribunal decision. This judgment may cause some reappraisal of the Government's plans in the Draft Mental Health Bill. In the meantime it sharpens the focus on the ASW's role.

A brief history of the developing role of the ASW can be found in Brown (2002).

ROLE OF THE APPROVED SOCIAL WORKER

There are various requirements of an ASW, which can be summarized as follows:

- To interview the patient in a 'suitable manner' (Section 13).
- To have 'regard to any wishes expressed by relatives' (Section 13).
- To consider 'all the circumstances of the case', including:
  - past history of the patient's mental disorder;
  - the patient's present condition;
  - social, family and personal factors;
  - the wishes of the patient and their relatives;
  - medical opinion (Memorandum).

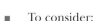

- To consider:
  - informal admission;
  - day care;
  - outpatient treatment;
  - community psychiatric nursing support;
  - crisis intervention centres;
  - primary healthcare support;
  - local authority social services provision;
  - support from friends, relatives and voluntary agencies (Memorandum).
- To decide whether 'detention in a hospital is in all the circumstances of the case the most appropriate way of providing the care and medical treatment of which the patient stands in need' (Section 13).
- To ensure that it is 'necessary or proper for the application to be made by' the ASW (Section 13).
- To take such steps as are practicable to inform the nearest relative that an application has been, or is about to be, made and inform them of their powers of discharge under Section 23 (Section 11).
- (If considering Section 3) to ensure that the nearest relative does not object to the application being made (Section 11).
- To convey the patient to hospital if an application is made by the ASW (with the powers of a constable) (Sections 6 and 137).
- If the ASW has been unable to inform the nearest relative before the patient's admission, then he or she should notify the hospital as soon as this has been done (Code of Practice).
- If the patient is admitted, then the ASW should make sure that any moveable property of the patient is protected (Section 48 National Assistance Act 1948).
- If the nearest relative applies for a Section 2 or Section 3, then a social worker must 'interview the patient and produce a report on his social circumstances' for the hospital managers (Section 14).
- If required to do so by the nearest relative, the social services department must direct an ASW to assess whether to make an application for detention. If the ASW does not apply, then the ASW must give his or her reasons in writing to the nearest relative (Section 13).
- To leave an outline report at the hospital when the patient is admitted, giving reasons for the admission and any practical matters about the patient's circumstances that the hospital should know (Code of Practice).

ASSESSMENT FOR POSSIBLE COMPULSORY ADMISSION OR GUARDIANSHIP

The key professionals in assessing a person's needs for possible compulsory admission to hospital, or for guardianship, are two doctors and an ASW. Although the nearest relative may apply for detention, the Code of Practice states at Paragraph 2.35 that the ASW is usually the correct applicant. In practice, nearest-relative applications are rare. The Mental Health Act 1983 sets out the criteria that must be satisfied before a person can be detained. These were considered in Chapter 3 of this book. This chapter will consider the process of assessment and the guidance contained in the Code of Practice. Chapter 2 of the Code of Practice covers assessment for possible admission. Although it makes some reference to guardianship, there is also further guidance on this in Chapter 13 of the Code. Chapter 2 was redrafted to bring together the material on professional communication, as this was seen as central to the process of assessment. The Code of Practice states:

> 2.3 Doctors and ASWs undertaking assessments need to apply professional judgement, and reach decisions, independently of each other but in a framework of co-operation and mutual support. Good working relationships require knowledge and understanding by the members of each profession of the other's distinct role and responsibilities. Unless there are good reasons for undertaking separate assessments, assessments should be carried out jointly by the ASW and doctor(s). It is essential that at least one of the doctors undertaking the medical assessment discusses the patient with the applicant (ASW or nearest relative) and desirable for both of them to do this.
>
> 2.4 Everyone involved in assessment should be alert to the need to provide support for colleagues, especially where there is a risk of the patient causing physical harm. Staff should be aware of circumstances where the police should be called to provide assistance, and how to use that assistance to minimise the risk of violence.

Paragraph 2.6 of the Code considers the statutory criteria that need to be satisfied before a patient is admitted under Part II of the Act. It also sets out a number of other factors that should be taken into consideration when making an assessment. These are:

- the guiding principles in Chapter 1;
- the patient's wishes and view of his or her own needs;
- the patient's social and family circumstances;
- the nature of the illness/behaviour disorder and its course;
- what may be known about the patient by his or her nearest relative, any other relatives or friends and professionals involved, assessing in particular how reliable this information is;
- other forms of care or treatment including, where relevant, consideration of whether the patient would be willing to accept medical treatment in hospital informally or as an out-patient and of whether guardianship would be appropriate …;
- the needs of the patient's family or others with whom he or she lives;
- the need for others to be protected from the patient;
- the burden on those close to the patient of a decision not to admit under the Act.

There are several guiding principles at Paragraph 1.1, including that people should:

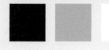

- be given respect for their qualities, abilities and diverse backgrounds as individuals and be assured that account will be taken of their age, gender, sexual orientation, social, cultural and religious background, but that general assumptions will not be made on the basis of any one of these characteristics;
- have their needs taken fully into account, though it is recognized that, within available resources, it may not always be practicable to meet them in full;
- be given any necessary treatment or care in the least controlled and segregated facilities compatible with ensuring their own health or safety or the safety of other people;
- be discharged from detention or other powers provided by the Act as soon as it is clear that their application is no longer justified.

Interpreters

Paragraph 1.4 of the Code states:

Local and Health Authorities and Trusts should ensure that ASWs, doctors, nurses and others receive sufficient guidance in the use of interpreters and should make arrangements for there to be an easily accessible pool of trained interpreters. Authorities and Trusts should consider co-operating in making this provision.

Section 13 of the Act requires the ASW to interview the patient in a 'suitable manner' and Paragraph 2.12 of the Code gives some detailed guidance on this. The Code balances the need for a full assessment with the risks to the worker, patient and others.

Nearest relative

The guidance in the Code on involving the nearest relative has been revised to take into account case experiences under the Act. This includes:

2.14 The ASW must attempt to identify the patient's nearest relative as defined in section 26 of the Act ... It is important to remember that the nearest relative for the purposes of the Act may not be the same person as the patient's 'next of kin', and also that the identity of the nearest relative is liable to change with the passage of time. The ASW must then ensure that the statutory obligations to the nearest relative set out in section 11 of the Act are fulfilled. In addition the ASW should where possible:
   a. ascertain the nearest relative's views about both the patient's needs and the relative's own needs in relation to the patient;
   b. inform the nearest relative of the reasons for considering an application for admission under the Mental Health Act and the effects of making such an application.
2.15 It is a statutory requirement to take such steps as are practicable to inform the nearest relative about an application for admission under

section 2 and of their power of discharge (section 11(3)). If the ASW has been unable to inform the nearest relative before the patient's admission he or she should notify the hospital as soon as this has been done.

2.16   Consultation by the ASW with the nearest relative about possible application for admission under section 3 or reception into guardianship is a statutory requirement unless it is not reasonably practicable or would involve unreasonable delay (section 11(4)). Circumstances in which the nearest relative need not be informed or consulted include those where the ASW cannot obtain sufficient information to establish the identity or location of the nearest relative or where to do so would require an excessive amount of investigation. Practicability refers to the availability of the nearest relative and not to the appropriateness of informing or consulting the person concerned. If the ASW has been unable to consult the nearest relative before making an application for admission for treatment (section 3) he or she should persist in seeking to contact the nearest relative so as to inform the latter of his or her powers to discharge the patient under section 23. The ASW should inform the hospital as soon as this has been done.

Delegation of nearest relative's functions

Paragraph 2.17 of the Code states:

> If the nearest relative would find it difficult to undertake the functions defined in the Act or is reluctant for any reason to do this Regulation 14 allows him or her to delegate those functions to another person. ASWs should consider proposing this in appropriate cases.

Paragraph 2.21 of the Code notes that when the ASW has reached a decision, he or she should tell (with reasons):

- the patient;
- the patient's nearest relative (whenever practicable);
- the doctor(s) involved in the assessment;
- the key worker, if the patient is on a care-programme approach (CPA);
- the patient's general practitioner (GP), if he or she was not involved in the assessment.

In cases in which a patient has been taken to a place of safety under Section 136 of the Act, the assessment by an ASW and doctor should begin as soon as possible after arrival at the place of safety. Local policies should set target times for the commencement of the assessment.

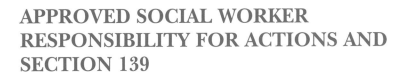

APPROVED SOCIAL WORKER RESPONSIBILITY FOR ACTIONS AND SECTION 139

There are a number of myths concerning the ASW's position in terms of responsibility for actions that they take under the Mental Health Act. For example, some people consider ASWs to be acting as free agents, with their employing authorities having no responsibility for their actions. Jones (2003, p. 96) clarifies this when he considers the ASW's position when deciding whether to make an application as per Section 13 of the Act:

> The duty is placed on the approved social worker and not on his employing authority. An approved social worker is therefore personally liable for his actions when carrying out functions under this Act. He should exercise his own judgement, based upon social and medical evidence, and not act at the behest of his employers, medical practitioners or other persons who might be involved with the patient's welfare.

Jones is also of the opinion that the ASW owes a duty of care to the people he or she is assessing for possible admission under the Act. ASWs should record the reasons for their decisions concerning applications. The general role of ASWs and how they are integrated within a mental health service is considered below.

Section 139 of the Mental Health Act is of importance when considering the liability of an ASW for actions taken in relation to the Act:

> 139(1) No person shall be liable, whether on the ground of want of jurisdiction or any other ground, to any civil or criminal proceedings to which he would have been liable apart from this section in respect of any act purporting to be done in pursuance of this Act or any regulations or rules made under this Act, or in, or in pursuance of anything done in, the discharge of functions conferred by any other enactment on the authority having jurisdiction under Part VII of this Act, unless the act was done in bad faith or without reasonable care.
>
> (2) No civil proceedings shall be brought against any person in any court in respect of any such act without the leave of the High Court; and no criminal proceedings shall be brought against any person in any court in respect of any such act except by or with the consent of the Director of Public Prosecutions.

This does not prevent the patient from applying to the High Court for a writ of Habeas Corpus so that the lawfulness of the detention can be tested.

Whether a person has acted in bad faith or without reasonable care is a question of fact, with the burden of proof lying with the applicant. The relevance of the Code of Practice to any action against an ASW can be seen in Paragraph 1 of the introduction to the Code, which states:

> The Act does not impose a legal duty to comply with the Code but, as it is a statutory document, failure to follow it could be referred to in evidence in legal proceedings.

As noted in Chapter 11, the Code's status has been enhanced by the Court of Appeal case of *R (on the application of Munjaz)* v. *Mersey Care NHS Trust* (2003), where the Court held that the Code must be followed unless there are good reasons for departing from it in relation to a particular patient.

A positive point of information for ASWs and employers is noted by Jones (2003, p. 439):

> Although an approved social worker acts in a personal capacity ... as an employee he will be protected by the doctrine of vicarious liability and the local authority will be liable for wrongs done by him while acting in the course of his employment. A legal action brought against either an approved social worker or his employing authority will succeed only if evidence of bad faith or lack of reasonable care is present (s139).

Hoggett (1996, p. 250) takes a critical stance on Section 139:

> ... there is no necessary connection between vexatiousness and the use of compulsion under the Mental Health Act. There is no evidence that the floodgates would open if section 139 were entirely repealed. There is more evidence, from a series of reports and investigations, that mental patients are in a peculiarly powerless position which merits, if anything, extra safeguards rather than the removal of those available to everyone else.

To act in good faith and reasonable care, we suggest that an ASW needs to be 'angst-ridden but strangely decisive', i.e. concerned to respect a person's right to freedom but prepared to intervene decisively when the level of mental disorder and risk requires it.

MANAGEMENT AND SUPERVISION OF APPROVED SOCIAL WORKERS

This part gives details of some key issues involved in the management and supervision of ASWs. It places the role of the ASW in context and clarifies which tasks can be performed only by an ASW. It also lists tasks that ASWs are likely to be involved in but that can also be performed by other staff.

Statutory basis for employing approved social workers

Section 114 of the Mental Health Act 1983 states the following:

114(1) A local social services authority shall appoint a sufficient number of approved social workers for the purpose of discharging the functions conferred on them by this Act.

(2) No person shall be appointed by a local social services authority as an approved social worker unless he is approved by the authority as having appropriate competence in dealing with persons who are suffering from mental disorder.

(3) In approving a person for appointment as an approved social worker a local social services authority shall have regard to such matters as the Secretary of State may direct.

The relevant circular, containing the Secretary of State's directions, is DHSS Circular Number LAC(86)15: *Mental Health Act 1983 – Approved Social Workers*. The Central Council for Education and Training in Social Work's (CCETSW) exercise of its powers given to it by the Secretary of State were initially set out in Paper 19:19. This was revised in 1993, and from spring 1995 all ASW training programmes have needed to assess specific competences. Before this, the responsibility for assessing the competence of ASWs was left exclusively with local authorities. Local authorities still retain a responsibility, as seen in Section 114 above, but the development of the new courses has probably led to more consistency across authorities in terms of standards.

The General Social Care Council (GSCC) has taken over responsibility for ASW programmes from the CCETSW. These ASW training programmes are now expected to be linked to universities, which will be seen increasingly to be responsible for standards of assessment. As an example, the current ASW training programmes in south London, south-west England and Hampshire have been approved by Bournemouth University for academic purposes and by the GSCC as conforming to revised regulations now set out in *Assuring Quality for Mental Health Social Work* (CCETSW 2000). The three programmes have adopted common assessment methods and have also had their ASW courses validated as part of a BA (Honours) programme (or postgraduate diploma for existing graduates) by Bournemouth University. On completion of the BA (or graduate diploma), candidates are awarded the GSCC's Postqualifying Award, as well as the Mental Health Social Work Award, which makes them eligible to be appointed by a local authority to practise as an ASW.

Role of approved social workers and their supervision and management needs

DHSS Circular Number LAC(86)15 states:

14. Approved social workers should have a wider role than reacting to requests for admission to hospital, making the necessary arrangements and ensuring compliance with the law. They should have the specialist knowledge and skills to make appropriate decisions in respect of both clients and their relatives and to gain the confidence of colleagues in the health services with whom they are required to collaborate. They must be familiar with the day to day working of an integrated mental health service and be able to assess what other services may be required and know how to mobilise them. They should have access to, consultation with and supervision from qualified and experienced senior officers. Their role is to prevent the necessity for compulsory admission to hospital as well as to make application where they decide this is appropriate.

Section 115 and Paragraph 2.11 of the Code of Practice require the ASW to have some form of identification. Ideally, this should be a sealed identity card and should include a photograph, name, local authority details and contact number, date of appointment as ASW and/or expiry date, and signature of director. Some authorities find it helpful to quote Section 115 rights of access on the reverse.

APPROVED SOCIAL WORKERS' TASKS

Sections 6 and 137: if an application is made, the ASW has the powers of a constable to convey the patient to hospital (see also Chapter 11 of the Code of Practice).

Section 8: an ASW may be asked to carry out the functions of guardian by the local authority.

*Section 11(3): the ASW should take such steps as are practicable to inform the nearest relative that an application has been, or is about to be, made and inform them of their powers of discharge under Section 23. This should include reference to the responsible medical officer's ability under Section 25 to block the discharge order if they consider the patient to be 'dangerous'.

*Section 11(4): if it is an application for admission for treatment or for guardianship, then the ASW must ensure that the nearest relative does not object to the application being made.

*Section 13(1): 'It shall be the duty of an approved social worker to make an application for admission to hospital or a guardianship application in respect of a patient within the area of the local social services authority by which that officer is appointed in any case where he is satisfied that such an application ought to be made and is of the opinion, having regard to any wishes expressed by relatives of the patient or any other relevant circumstances, that it is necessary or proper for the application to be made by him.' In carrying out this task, the ASW must interview the patient in a 'suitable manner' and consider 'all the circumstances of the case', including past history of the patient's mental disorder; the patient's present condition; the effect on this of any social, family and personal factors; the wishes of the patient; and medical opinion. The ASW should consider informal admission, day care, outpatient treatment, community psychiatric nursing support, crisis intervention centres, primary healthcare support, social services provision, friends, relatives and voluntary agencies. The ASW must then decide whether 'detention in a hospital is in all the circumstances of the case the most appropriate way of providing the care and medical treatment of which the patient stands in need' (Section 13(2)). Although it is important to stress that the ASW is acting as an officer of the local authority who is accountable for the ASW's actions, it should be noted that the ASW also carries a personal responsibility in making this decision.

Section 13(4): if required to do so by the nearest relative, the social services department must direct an ASW to assess whether to make an application for detention.

*Section 13(4): if the ASW does not apply, he or she must give reasons in writing to the nearest relative.

Section 14: if the nearest relative applies for section 2 or 3, a social worker must 'interview the patient and produce a report on his social circumstances' for the hospital managers.

*Section 25B: where appropriate and having regard to the patient's history, the ASW must provide a written recommendation in the prescribed form for supervised discharge.

*Section 29: in certain circumstances, the ASW must apply to the County Court for the displacement and/or appointment of a nearest relative for the patient.

*Section 115: the ASW must enter and inspect premises where there is reasonable cause to believe that a patient is not under proper care.

*Section 135: the ASW must apply for a warrant to search for and remove to a place of safety patients or persons living alone or in need of care.

Section 136: the ASW must interview a person arrested by the police under Section 136.

Section 48 of National Assistance Act 1948: if a patient is admitted to hospital or Part III (of the National Assistance Act 1948) accommodation, then the local authority must ensure that any moveable property of the patient is protected.

*Tasks marked with an asterisk can be performed only within the local authority by an ASW.

REFERENCES

Brown, R (2002). A response to the Draft Mental Health Bill. *Journal of Mental Health Law* **8**, 392–8.

CCETSW (2000). *Assuring Quality for Mental Health Social Work.* London: Central Council for Education and Training in Social Work.

Department of Health (1998). *Mental Health Act 1983: Memorandum on Parts I to VI, VIII and X.* London: HMSO.

Hoggett, B (1996). *Mental Health Law,* 4th edn. London: Sweet and Maxwell.

Jones, R (2003). *Mental Health Act Manual,* 8th edn. London: Sweet & Maxwell.

Assessment of risk of violence

INTRODUCTION

Violence has multifactorial causes and is a biopsychosocial environmental phenomenon. Clearly all behaviour has a biochemical basis, but while biochemical abnormalities can cause psychological symptoms, including aggression, there is also increasing evidence that psychological events, e.g. severe abuse in childhood or severe psychological trauma in adulthood, may cause neurobiological abnormalities, e.g. in serotonin (5-hydroxytryptamine, 5-HT) metabolism in adults. Models of violence are shown in Table 15.1. No model can explain adequately all violence, and some models are more appropriate than others for different situations.

Aggression

Aggression, using the biological definition, is intraspecific fighting. Normal aggression is seen in all members of a species, while pathological aggression or violence is either excessive in degree and/or arises from mental disorder. Almost all forms of mental disorder can be associated with pathological aggression and violence (Table 15.2), although anyone can become violent. There has been debate about whether aggression is instinct, i.e. determined genetically but called out by the environment, or learned. Probably there is a normal inborn assertiveness, with aggression being secondary to early developmental deprivation and insults and/or mental disorder, rather than a primary drive. Aggression often follows frustration and threat, e.g. to a low self-esteem, and increasing tension. Aggression may, of course, be displaced from the original object on to a symbolic representation of it, e.g. arson, or anger towards the person's mother displaced on to women in general. Aggression can also be a social phenomena, e.g. in altruistic aggression and war.

Violence, dangerousness and risk

Violence is action; dangerousness is a potential and a matter of opinion. The term 'risk' is now being used increasingly in professional practice in preference to the term 'dangerousness'. Risk is, ideally, a matter of statistical fact. It emphasizes a continuum of levels of risk, varying not only with the individual but also with the

TABLE 15.1 Models and putative causative factors of violence

Biological factors	Fight or flight response
	Males and young people more violent
	Testosterone levels
	Reduced serotonin (5-HT) levels in brain
Alcohol, drugs	50 per cent of violent offences follow alcohol abuse in the UK
	Disinhibition
Psychological models	
Instrumental aggression	Learn to achieve ends by violence
Cognitive model	Look at world aggressively
Behavioural model	Inconsistent, erratic parental punishment
Social learning	Peer pressure/modelling (Bandura)
Status	Status of being violent
Psychodynamic models	
Freudian	Primary drive due to frustration
	Later, primary drive libido, aggression secondary drive
Kleinian	Annihilation anxiety
Kohut	Secondary to developmental insults or deprivations
Object relation school (Winnicott)	Aggression is creative of another
Attachment theory	Insecurely attached infant, e.g. deprived or abused, relates to others with hostility
Family factors	Physical abuse as child
	Parental discord and violence
	Parental irritability, usually due to depression
Social models	Subcultural norm, e.g. Hells Angels
	Pub brawls
	Sporting, political and industrial violence
	Relative poverty and inequality
	Comparative anthropology, e.g. Mead's studies
Environmental factors	Avoidance of frustration by well-structured and staffed milieu and non-provocative regime

context. It may change over time and, in principle, should be based on objective assessment. Dangerousness tends to imply an all-or-nothing phenomenon and a static characteristic of an individual. However, clearly risk assessment is less important than risk management, although risk management does not imply risk elimination.

Risk assessed as low, medium, high or very high is often arbitrary. The meaning of risk can include:

■ likelihood of offending: risk measures are often over periods of 20 years;
■ immediacy of offending: risk instruments say nothing about this;

TABLE 15.2 Violence and psychiatric disorder

Non-psychiatric causes: social

Economic

Criminal, e.g. drug dealing

Cultural, e.g. subcultures

Psychiatric causes

Violence or threats of violence in 40% pre-admission

Schizophrenia: paranoid and non-paranoid

Mania, hypomania but also depression

Alcohol abuse and withdrawal

Drug abuse and withdrawal

     Hallucinogens, e.g. phencyclidine (PCP)

     Benzodiazepine withdrawal

Organic mental disorder and brain damage, epilepsy (especially temporal lobe epilepsy), dementia

Personality disorder, particularly antisocial, impulsive and borderline

Learning disability

Child and adolescent behaviour disorders

Post-traumatic stress disorder

Dissociative states

Intrafamilial

Spousal abuse

Child abuse

Elder abuse

- frequency of offending: sadistic murderers rarely kill again;
- consequences of offending: exhibitionists are at high risk but have low consequences.

For instance, what does an 80 per cent chance of offending mean? Is it eight out of ten individuals like this person will offend, or, given the same circumstances, that this person will offend eight out of ten times? Is 80 per cent merely a measure of subjective belief?

Background to risk assessment

Risk assessment developed from observations on released prisoners, empirical associations with reconviction and its extension to forensic psychiatric patients. The Ritchie (1994) report of inquiry into the care and treatment of Christopher Clunis, who 'avoidably' killed Jonathan Zito, identified failures in risk assessment and risk management and inadequacies in communication and service provision. Christopher Clunis was given 20 different clinical diagnoses, was placed in about

20 different accommodations, and was seen by about 35 different professionals in the period before the offence.

In response to increasing public concern that something needed to be done to improve the management of people, albeit few in number, who are deemed at serious risk to others, e.g. predatory paedophiles, legislation has been introduced to improve the risk management of such individuals. This includes the Sex Offenders Act 1997, the Crime Sentences Act 1997, the Criminal Justice and Court Services Act 2000 and Multi-Agency Public Protection Panels and Arrangements (MAPPS or MAPPAS) (2001).

Ethics of risk assessment

Ethical issues in risk assessment include whether it can be done adequately and, if so, whether it should be undertaken if no treatment is available and it may thus merely increase the length of a custodial sentence. Risk assessment can be stigmatizing. Further questions include whether it should be undertaken on every psychiatric patient or at least every forensic psychiatric patient seen. For psychiatry, key issues are what the risk is and whether it can be modified. However, evaluating whether residual risk is acceptable may be a matter for society, Mental Health Review Tribunals and potential victims.

VIOLENCE AND MENTAL ILLNESS

There is no evidence of increasing rates of homicide by mentally ill people in the UK (Bennett 1996, Taylor and Gunn 1999), in spite of this being the media and the public's perception, which probably reflects only increasing awareness. Such homicides by mentally ill people have a negligible effect on public safety compared with other factors, such as road-traffic accidents. In the past, factors associated with violence were said to be the same, regardless of whether the offender was mentally ill, e.g. personality disorder, impulsivity, anger, violent family background and substance abuse. However, since 1992, studies have shown that having a diagnosis of mental illness is associated weakly with violence due to a subgroup with specific types of symptoms such as paranoid (persecutory) delusions (false beliefs) and delusions of passivity (being under external control). It is thus certain symptoms, and not a particular psychiatric diagnosis alone, that are associated with violence. Nevertheless, the risk of violence is still better predicted by being a young male than by having a diagnosis of schizophrenia (Swanson et al. 1990).

Psychiatrists are better than chance or lay people in predicting violence and better still at assessing situations where there is no risk. However, they tend to underestimate the risk of violence in females (Lidz et al. 1993). Professionals also underestimate the high background base rates of violence in the community in general, e.g. up to 40 per cent of males may have been seriously violent by the age of 32 years (Farrington 1995). The majority of violence never results in criminal charges. This also applies to inpatients who are violent, where formal charges may often be seen as serving little purpose if the patient is to remain in hospital.

Among individuals with mental illness, affective disorders are under-represented in forensic psychiatric facilities. Violence is, however, increased in people with schizophrenia, especially those who have drifted out of treatment, and in young males with acute schizophrenia compared with those with chronic schizophrenia. Violence may arise directly from positive symptoms of mental illness, such as delusions (false beliefs) and hallucinations (e.g. voices). Mental illness, especially schizophrenia, may, however, lead indirectly to violence through associated deterioration in social functioning and personality, so that such individuals become more antisocial and impulsive and with a lower tolerance to stress. This sometimes leads to disputes in court about the disposal of such individuals with few or no positive psychotic symptoms, with such individuals sometimes being given, wrongly, an additional diagnosis of personality disorder to explain their violence. A mentally ill individual may also behave violently for 'normal' emotional reasons, such as fear and anger, and then experience accompanying corresponding psychotic symptoms, e.g. hallucinations of aggressive content. Violence, law involvement and imprisonment may themselves precipitate mental illness.

For a mentally ill person, a key issue is whether the individual has a delusion of a content on which he or she might act dangerously, e.g. of persecution or infidelity, but even then not all morbidly jealous individuals, for instance, assault their spouse. Twenty per cent of people presenting to hospital with their first episode of schizophrenia have threatened the lives of others, but among these half have already been ill for a year (Humphreys et al. 1992). Overall, however, it is unusual for a person with schizophrenia to present for the first time with serious violence. One established period of higher risk is within a few months of discharge from hospital (Taylor 1993). People with both schizophrenia and substance abuse have higher rates of violence than those with substance abuse alone, who, in turn, have higher rates than those with schizophrenia alone (Swanson et al. 1990).

In countries with high homicide rates, such as the USA, this is usually due to high numbers of non-mentally ill offenders, their violence being related to criminal activities, drug dealing and cultural and economic factors, and there is a lower proportion of mentally ill homicide offenders. Rates of mentally ill homicide offenders may be fairly constant across countries.

Research has shown a consistent association between violence and delusions, particularly of threat/control override content, e.g. persecutory delusions, passivity delusions and thought insertion (Link and Stueve 1994). These findings are in keeping with the social psychology theory that violence in general is associated with an individual feeling under threat or losing control of his or her situation.

Based particularly on the work of Steadman and Monahan's group (Steadman et al. 1998) in the USA (the McArthur Foundation Violence Risk Assessment Study), the Royal College of Psychiatrists in 1996, in their booklet *Assessment and Clinical Management of Risk of Harm to Other People*, detailed 'warning signs' that professionals should be aware of. These were:

- beliefs of persecution, or control by external forces;
- previous violence or suicide attempts;
- social restlessness;
- poor compliance with medication or treatment;
- substance abuse;

- hostility, suspiciousness and anger;
- threats.

Steadman and colleagues (2000) have developed a computer algorithm for risk assessment of violence (not homicide) (the Monahan/Steadman iterative classification tree).

Psychiatric patients tend to peak for violent offending at a later age than the general population. It is important to be aware that the oft-quoted 'best predictor of future behaviour is past behaviour' is based on non-psychiatric populations and, in any case, accounts for only five per cent of the variance. A history of previous violence is, of course, required for this to be relevant in any case. Among severely (psychotic) mentally ill people, delusions of threat/control override are better predictors than past behaviour.

Among all individuals, including mentally ill people, a history of expressed threats (as opposed to generalized anger), substance misuse and a history of personal deprivation and/or abuse are all associated with violence. Law-breaking behaviour in general and violence in particular usually decrease when the basic needs of an individual are met. For instance, an individual with schizophrenia who is violent often has a characteristic history of not only non-compliance with medication, leading to relapse of his or her mental illness, but also of being in a situation of social isolation and poor home conditions. Some individuals may even offend to remove themselves from their situation in the community to the security of prison or hospital. The risk of self-harm or suicide is greater for people with schizophrenia, even if they have behaved seriously violently, than homicide or serious harm to others. Compulsory admission under the Mental Health Act for reasons of a patient's health is clearly better than at a later time for the protection of others as a last resort after someone has been hurt.

In summary, the existing evidence suggests that there is a link between mental illness and violence. Mental illness is a risk factor, but not a large one, and the risk is increased by substance abuse.

RISK ASSESSMENT

This can be only a probability assessment. Dangerous behaviour is rare and sporadic, so most of our worries about individuals never materialize. This can lull professionals into a false sense of security and to underestimate the risk. Risk assessment can be difficult, e.g. predicting how an individual in conditions of security will behave outside such conditions with the availability of alcohol and illicit drugs and potential victims, or predicting intrafamilial violence among those with personality disorder.

When undertaking a risk assessment, it is necessary to look at factors not only in the individual but also in his or her victims or potential victims and the environment, including the security of interview rooms and procedures for assessing an individual in the community, i.e. the offence is a function of the offender, the victim and the environment.

Dangerousness is often associated with repetition, failure to respond to the counter-measures of society, unpredictability and untreatability. Truly dangerous people are, by definition, unpredictable. People labelled at risk of serious harm to others include those previously convicted of dangerous offences, those who use firearms and other weapons and, by definition, people subject to restrictions under Section 41 of the Mental Health Act 1983 and those in special hospitals. A legal offence category may not reflect the current risk. Short-term prediction is better than long-term prediction; the risk of serious harm itself is often long-term and not obvious on short-term follow-up. False-positive assessments of risk are made more often than false-negative assessments. Professionals tend to err on the side of caution, but they may be reluctant to take on individuals considered at serious risk of harming others due to negative counter-transference feelings, e.g. related to shock at past offences or from fear of being held professionally responsible for the individual's actions and feeling overwhelmed by this. This in turn can lead to overestimating risks and inappropriate precipitate actions to cover oneself and displace responsibility on to others. The courts, however, expect professionals to give an opinion on dangerousness. On occasions, professionals inappropriately attempt to 'rescue' dangerous untreatable individuals who they feel have been managed badly by others. Professionals must guard against overidentifying with the subject, denying what they do not wish to hear and not acting on threats and behaviour giving rise to concern, especially among those in the community who, if they had been inpatients and behaved in such a fashion, would cause great concern. Professionals must ask directly what thoughts, fantasies, impulses and/or plans to be violent an individual has, e.g. of homicide, in a manner that they would question directly in a suicide risk assessment.

Risk factors include dispositional factors, such as demographic factors, historical factors, including past violence, constitutional factors, including stress and social support, and clinical factors, including diagnoses, symptoms and substance abuse. A summary of variables often sought in risk assessment includes the following:

- demographic factors, e.g. previous violence, age, sex. Such variables can be documented easily. Among mentally ill people, age under 35 years and male predominance are less predictive. Risk in females is underrated (Lidz et al. 1993). The relationship of violence to when the person is mentally unwell is of importance;
- environmental factors: these are harder to document and include family support, poor social network, lack of intimate relationships, unemployment, poverty and homelessness, and availability of weapons;
- substance abuse: alcohol and cannabis abuse are most common;
- current context: recent major life events, e.g. loss;
- dispositional factors, e.g. impulsivity, irritability, suspiciousness;
- interests, e.g. cruelty, fantasies, weapons;
- social functioning;
- attitudes, e.g. to violence and previous and future victims;
- poor engagement and compliance with services;
- mental state, e.g. feelings, emotions, thinking, perception, behaviour. Violence is associated with fear, anger, humiliation and jealousy. Note should be made of tension, depression, paranoid ideas, delusions, hallucinations, including command hallucinations, clouding of consciousness and confusion, and anger and threats. Data on command hallucinations are equivocal but more positive for threat/control override

delusional symptoms (Link and Stueve 1994), e.g. paranoid delusions and delusions of passivity.

Table 15.3 shows the factors to be considered in a risk assessment with special reference to an offender.

TABLE 15.3 Risk assessment

The aim is to get an understanding of the risk from a detailed historical longitudinal overview, obtaining information not only from the patient, who may minimize his or her past history, but from informants. Ideally, it should not be a one-off single-interview assessment.

1 *Reconstruct in detail what happened at the time of the offence or behaviour causing concern.* Independent information from statements of victims or witnesses or police records should be obtained where available. Do not rely on what the offender tells you or the legal offence category, e.g. arson may be of a wastepaper bin in a busy ward or with an intent to kill. Possession of an offensive weapon may have been a prelude to homicide.
Offence = Offender × Victim × Circumstances/Environment

(i) *Offender:*
– alone or in group, e.g. gang (less inhibition in groups);
– planned or impulsive (beware rationalization of behaviour post-offence);
– triggers, e.g., behavioural, emotional, physiological or situational;
– provoked;
– displaced aggression, e.g. mother kills baby to spite father;
– recent discontinuation of medication;
– disruption of therapeutic alliance, e.g. professional holidays;
– during other criminal behaviour or deliberate self-harm.

Mental state at time of offence: link specific symptoms, e.g. delusions, or emotional state, e.g. overarousal, anxiety, fear, irritability, anger or suspiciousness, or disinhibition, to violence.
Degree and quality of violence: overall more violent, more risk. Bizarre violence seen in mental illness and severe psychopathic disorder. Is there satisfaction from inflicting pain? The more precarious the psychological defences, the more violence. More often not predictive of repetition, but reflects relationship with victim, e.g. resistance of victim to dying and arousal of offender. Parodoxically, less violence in general if victim fights back, except in rape and sexual assaults, where violence may increase.
Alcohol/drugs facilitating or precipitating aggression.
Use of weapons, e.g. carrying means of destruction, if only for self-protection, e.g. knife, if loses temper.

(ii) *Victim:*
– Victim may be consciously or unconsciously provocative, e.g. if drunk, due to their own background, or if not aware of effect of own behaviour on others.
– Is violence against a particular named individual for specific reasons, e.g. relative, therapist or victim blamed in homosexual panic, against a

particular type of victim, or against staff with whom in clinical contact, all staff of an institution, or the world in general?
– Is victim merely an object of displaced aggression to others, e.g. from mother, society?
– Is victim the real intended victim? If not, risk of repetition.

(iii) *Circumstances/environment:*
– Current stresses, particularly recent loss or threat of loss events.
– Circumstances, e.g. both offender and victim intoxicated in a public house.
– Precipitating factors in social environment. Now removed? Can they be modified?
– Culture: inhibiting or sensitizing? Varies over time.

(iv) *Type of offence behaviour:*
Was offence without warning or could it have been predicted? What caused it to cease?
Some behaviours are predictive of future dangerousness, including:
– morbid jealousy;
– sadistic murder;
– sexual offender overwhelmed with aggression;
– at least two offences of serious violence or sexual assault.

2 *Behaviour after offence:*
– did the offender summon help for victim?
– freezing;
– regression: associated with future dangerousness;
– manner of talking about the offence, e.g. dispassionate, guilt-free manner or capacity for sympathetic identification. Any 'unfinished business'?
– admission of guilt and transparency;
– beware protective psychological defence mechanisms, e.g. after homicide, leading to appearance of callous indifference.

3 *Progress in custody and/or hospital:*
– capacity for self-control or explosiveness;
– no relationships;
– feelings of professionals, especially females, in cases of psychopaths and sex offenders;
– reaction of other inmates/patients;
– do his or her pets survive?

4 *At interview (ideally, interview and mental state examination should take place on more than one occasion and should be repeated over time):*
– threats of violence (verbal anger is a poor predictor of violence);
– expressed intent;
– feeling of fear in interviewer;
– impulsive: cannot delay gratification;
– paucity of feeling for victim/indifference;
– over- or undercontrolled;
– depression;
– morbid jealousy;

– content of delusions, hallucinations, etc., e.g. threat/control override, i.e. of paranoid or passivity content;
– insight into mental disorder and offending: is violence regarded as unacceptable?
– attempting to self-control? Help requested?

5   *Assessment of personality traits:*
– informants and historical information important, especially when offender mentally ill;
– impulsive, antisocial, lack of guilt, affectionless;
– deceptive/lying (e.g. due to learned strategy to deal with overdominant or aggressive parents) compared with transparent;
– inadequate personalities overall commit more serious offences than aggressive psychopaths;
– jealous/paranoid: does he or she feel continually threatened?
– poor self-image, low self-esteem;
– over-/undercontrolled;
– features of Brittain's sadistic murderer syndrome (see his or her room contents, e.g. weapons, Nazi gear);
– how does he or she handle stress, e.g. if by violence, is this egosyntonic or egodystonic?
– formal psychometric testing of personality and intelligence may assist.

6   *Life history:*
Age: younger more dangerous than older (dangerousness generally decreases with age, except for sadists and offences of retaliation against women).
Sex: male more than female, except in psychiatric hospitals, where rates are similar.
Family history: deprived, neglect, physical and/or sexual parental abuse, alcoholic father, domineering mother, parental discord and violence.
Childhood: classic dangerous triad of enuresis, cruelty to animals and firesetting, although only cruelty to animals demonstrated to be predictive of future violence. Conduct disorder. A bully or bullied.
Employment: butchering, work in abattoir or for veterinary surgery, e.g. animals die in their care. Inability to sustain employment, e.g. due to problems of impulsivity or with authority or routine.
Sexual history: if sexual offence and no previous relationships with women, assume attacks will go on. Previous victimization. Sadistic or violent sexual thoughts, fantasies, impulses or behaviour.
Social restlessness: for example, frequent change of address or employment. Few relationships. Among groups where increased violence, e.g. homeless.
Previous medical history: head injury, brain damage (even minimal), temporal lobe epilepsy, extra Y chromosome. Abnormalities of electroencephalogram (EEG) or brain scans.
Substance abuse history.
Previous psychiatric history: diagnosis of psychopathy. Alcoholism or drug dependency. Low intelligence level. Previous suicidal behaviour, especially if impulsive and/or violent and/or associated with risk to others.

> *Relationship of offending to mental illness and its control by medication*, etc.
> Compliance with treatment, especially medication.
> *Attitudes to treatment.*
> *Previous forensic history:*
> – violent/non-violent;
> – worse if early-onset, persistent and serious;
> – ask how close to violence he or she comes and his or her most violent act in the past;
> – when is violence most likely to happen? Learn from 'near-misses';
> – any *evidence of escalation?*
> *Current support systems.*

Risk may change rapidly over time. If risk is identified, then it must be managed and the management plans documented. However, concern may arise before a non-cooperative patient is detainable under the Mental Health Act. Interventions may also increase the risk temporarily, e.g. following detention in hospital or enforced medication treatment. Whatever is done may not remove the entire risk. There is also the question of how many false positives of those deemed at risk are acceptable compared, for instance, with the price of one homicide. Serious harm often follows a sequence of decisions by professionals rather than one major error of judgement. There is also not much relationship between inpatient and outpatient violence.

Clinical or practical risk assessment

Risk assessment requires information gathering, including by a full history from the subject, examination of past records and/or statements when available in Crown Court criminal cases, and from informants, including arresting police officers. As a minimum, a risk assessment and management plan should include the following:

- Ask informants about history of violence.
- Request previous summaries, e.g. of inpatient care, and past psychiatric and probation reports.
- Document the above, and keep and use proper records.
- Make plans to manage the risk, and document this.
- Be particularly cautious in cases where treatment is refused, is reduced or is being withheld.

Clinical risk assessment, however, is unstructured, is usually biased by a few factors, is subject to subjective bias, sometimes is based on the last case seen that went wrong, shows poor consistency, is difficult to quantify, and is inductive, i.e. based on previous cases. There is no evidence that counter-transference is predictive.

Standardized structured risk-assessment instruments

Increasingly, clinical or practical risk assessment, involving consideration of the history, mental state and environment, is being supplemented by standardized actuarial and/or dynamic risk-assessment instruments, the latter alone often being insufficient. Thus, risk assessment = clinical assessment + standardized instrument assessment.

Structured risk assessments can be used merely as aide-memoires and reference points rather than being scored numerically. The lack of standardized assessments has been cited as a factor in the excess of females and people of Afro-Caribbean origin in special hospitals.

Structured risk assessments are more useful at high levels of risk but are not very useful in predicting isolated dangerous acts such as homicide. They are more useful in those diagnosed with personality disorders than psychoses and are also useful in predicting sex offending. Reliability is better with static rather than dynamic variables and hence less helpful in deciding on discharge. Some structured assessments may, however, record risk factors that are otherwise explainable clinically, e.g. lack of emotional expression may result from antipsychotic medication treatment.

Actuarial risk-assessment instruments

Actuarial risk-assessment instruments tend to measure static factors. Examples include the Violence Risk Appraisal Guide (VRAG) (Harris et al. 1993; Quinsey et al. 1998) and, for sex offenders, from the work of Hanson and Thornton (1999, 2000), Static 99 and the Risk Matrix 2000. Police use the Risk Matrix 2000 as a screen for cases referred to the MAPPS. Risk factors in this instrument include being male, younger age groups, and number of times in court for violent or sexual offences. The risk identified, however, is over a prolonged period. Actuarial risk-assessment instruments are objective, unbiased and deductive. While good at identifying low risk, they tend to overjudge high-risk cases. Problems with actuarial risk-assessment instruments include the facts that first-time offenders score low, they are poor predictors of young and female offenders, they are blind to current circumstances, e.g. a paedophile married to a female with children, and they provide a lifetime rather than an immediate assessment of risk.

Dynamic risk-assessment instruments

Dynamic risk-assessment instruments look at not only dynamic factors but frequently also actuarial factors.

The **Historical/Clinical/Risk Management 20-Item instrument (HCR-20)** (Webster et al. 1977) includes historical factors, present clinical factors and risk-management factors. Present clinical factors include insight, negative attitudes, active symptoms of major mental illness, impulsivity and unresponsiveness to treatment. Risk-management factors include future plans lacking feasibility, exposure to destabilizers, lack of personal support, non-compliance and stress. This instrument can be used as an enquiry guide and prompt rather than as a numerical rating scale. In some countries, its use is becoming mandatory for particular groups of serious offenders.

Hare's Psychopathy Checklist – Revised (PCL-R) (Hare 1991) has two main components: (i) emotional/interpersonal traits (Factor 1), such as callousness, selfishness and remorseless use of others, which are mainly static traits, and (ii) social deviance (Factor 2), i.e. chronically unstable and antisocial lifestyle, which has some dynamic elements and may vary between countries. It involves a structured interview and an expert rating form. It is for use in people aged 18 years or older. Items are scored on a three-point scale. Scores range from zero to 40. Only one-third of people with antisocial personality disorder reach the scale's criteria for psychopathy (i.e. score over 30). Some argue that such tools are superior to clinical risk assessment in people with personality disorder, while the reverse may be the case for people who are mentally ill. Candidates for dangerous severe personality disorder (DSPD) units are defined as having more than a 50 per cent risk of committing a serious offence due to a severe personality disorder, and the PCL-R is usually used preadmission, including to establish this risk.

The PCL-R has been supplemented by a 12-item screening version (PCL-SV) (Hart et al. 1995). Scores on this range from zero to 24 (cut-off 18) and have been found to have good predictive validity for violence (Monahan et al. 2000).

The most recent revision to the PCL-R is the PCL-R™ second edition (Hare 2003). This has a 20-item symptom–construct rating scale with a Quickscore Form to record and profile results. It subdivides both Factor 1 and Factor 2 into two valid subscales. Factor 1 is divided into Factor 1a Interpersonal (four items) and Factor 1b Affective (four items); Factor 2 is divided into Factor 2a Impulsive Lifestyle (five items) and Factor 2b Antisocial Behaviour (five items).

Other dynamic risk-assessment instruments include the Sexual Violence Risk Scale (SVR-20) (Boer et al. 1997), the Spousal Assault Risk Assessment Guide (SARA) (Kropp et al. 1995) and the Sex Offender Risk Appraisal Guide (SORAG) (Quinsey et al. 1995, 1998), a variation on the VRAG. The Structured Risk Assessment (SRA) framework developed by Hanson and Thornton (2000) for sex offenders now uses both the Risk Matrix 2000, based on static actuarial factors, and dynamic risk factors.

The Violence Risk Scale (VRS) was developed by Wong and Gordon (2000). This has been found to be particularly useful in the assessment of sex offenders, and it can measure change. It includes six static variables, including age and age at first conviction, and 20 dynamic variables, including violent lifestyle, criminal personality, mental disorder, substance misuse, community relationships, community supervision, release to a high-risk situation and anger and violence.

Actuarial variables should not override clinical variables, as the latter are more likely to determine when and how a person may behave dangerously. Uncertainty in risk assessment is due to the many variables involved, randomness, and the effects of human interaction and intervention. Dynamic variables are, by definition, subject to change and may be subject to interaction with other factors, such as other people, which actuarial risk assessments are generally less helpful in predicting. The situation is comparable to weather forecasting, which may be accurate in the short term and also, broadly, in the longer term, e.g. winter compared with summer, but not specific enough to indicate where it might rain in a few days' time. Structured risk assessments may provide evidence for institutionalizing a person, but they are less useful in deciding when to release a person from an institution.

Other problems in risk assessment include the following:

- The low base rate problem. For example, a rate of less than one per cent for serious violence makes it difficult to predict such a rare event.
- Risk valuation following risk assessment estimation. For example, what action is warranted by a particular risk of violence? What is an acceptable false-positive rate, e.g. for detaining patients?
- The quality of a professional's relationship with a patient determines the accuracy of a risk assessment, but admission to secure forensic psychiatric facilities often depends on bed availability. In contrast, mental state examination may be of little use in assessing risk of sex offending.
- Assessment scales have not always been developed in the populations to which they are applied, e.g. scales developed for non-psychiatric prison populations are used for psychiatric cases.

Risk assessment allows for a longitudinal formulation of the individual, assessment of whether any risk is unconditional or conditional on particular factors, and assessment of whether these factors are amenable to change. The aim should be to produce a person-specific biography of the individual, allowing the individual to tell his or her own story, and then to negotiate a plan of action with the individual and other parties. Risk assessment for violence has many parallels with suicide risk assessment.

RISK MANAGEMENT

Once a risk assessment is made, it is essential to develop and document a risk-management plan. In the community, careful supervision by well-briefed professionals is required. It is important not to ignore threats and to avoid provoking violence by appearing to precipitously reject requests for help. For an individual who has offended dangerously, a Mental Health Act 1983 Section 41 restriction order may need to be recommended to a Crown Court judge for the judge to add this to a Section 37 hospital order to 'protect the public from serious harm' and to facilitate long-term psychiatric management, including in the community, particularly with regard to compliance with treatment there but also by specifying a suitable place of residence. The Advisory Board on Restricted Patients (the Aarvold Committee) is appointed by the Home Secretary to advise him and to review restricted cases referred by him before conditional or absolute discharge. Between 15 and 20 per cent of restricted patients are so considered. Special hospital placement may be required if an individual suffers from a mental disorder and is a 'grave and immediate danger' to others, especially if the person is also at risk of determined absconding. A medium-secure unit may be indicated if a mentally disordered individual needs conditions of security that are less than those of a special hospital but are more than those of an ordinary locked intensive-care or low secure unit.

INQUIRIES INTO HOMICIDES BY PSYCHIATRIC PATIENTS

These are mandatory and have emphasized failures in care due to poor communication between professionals and agencies, downgrading of previous violence, failure to recognize and manage social restlessness and escalating problems, lack of contact of subjects with consultant psychiatrists, rigid catchment area practice, lack of resources, e.g. lack of acute beds and trained staff, failure to use the Mental Health Act appropriately to detain for reasons of health before violence occurs, and lack of carer involvement, although the latter may raise issues of patient confidentiality. Non-compliance with treatment in the community has been perhaps the most common major factor characterizing these cases. However, there can, of course, be no real 'supervision' in the community in the sense of continual observation. Overall, such inquiries have highlighted not the limitations of risk assessment, as real as these are, but failure to communicate or manage a known risk. Improving community psychiatric care may thus be more useful in reducing the risk of violence than attempts at perfecting risk-assessment instruments. Certainly, the use of standardized structured risk-assessment instruments would not alone prevent most homicides by psychiatric patients.

GOVERNMENT RESPONSES TO INQUIRY FINDINGS

The political pressure of 'something must be done' has led to the following:

- care-programme approach (CPA) (Department of Health 1990);
- supervision registers (NHS Management Executive 1994a);
- guidance on discharge of mentally disordered people (NHS Management Executive 1994b);
- Mental Health (Patients in the Community) Act 1995 (supervised discharge order).

The usefulness of the above measures remains open to question. The CPA is a process rather than a treatment; individuals may be unable or unwilling to comply, and families may or may not wish to be involved. On the positive side, the CPA is a needs-led multidisciplinary approach to developing a care plan, which has to be monitored and should always include a risk assessment. Drawbacks to the CPA include lack of resources, large caseloads, increase in time required for meetings and documentation, and it leading to defensive practice.

These government responses also occur against a background of a general decline in psychiatric hospital beds, e.g. from 152 000 in 1954 to 53 700 in 1993. Those psychiatric patients who have been violent in the community, however, tend not to be those who might previously have been on long-stay wards. However, if 100 long-term hospital beds are closed, then there is an additional need for about ten new acute beds to cope with resulting revolving-door admissions, and this can lead to a lack of acute beds for the emergency admission of violent patients. Increasing the number of hospital beds alone is not the whole solution, as there is also a need for other measures, such as short-term crisis community facilities. While inquiries emphasize the need for direct face-to-face contact between professionals and patients, an average inner-city caseload for a social worker is 20 and for a consultant psychiatrist 450–500, with 300 new patients a year; however, CPA arrangements technically are required for all patients and a legal duty of care applies to any patient to whom a professional talks. Funding also has not been related to epidemiology, e.g. in urban areas, where there is an excess of schizophrenia due to social drift, and where drug abuse and a younger population are also more evident, and there has otherwise been increased identification of cases, including via court and prison diversion schemes. One response by clinicians has been to increase the rates of detention under the Mental Health Act 1983, which has been most pronounced for Section 3 and for mental illness. While there has been no significant change in the number of Section 37 hospital orders, there has been an increase in Section 41 restriction orders. Another response has been the development of assertive outreach programmes.

Proactive measures to manage violence include adequate training of community mental health teams and the development of protocols for potential violent scenarios in hospital and in the community, e.g. for home visits. Risk assessment also should lead to the identification of warning signs indicating early signs of relapse or increased risk. The importance of communication between a general practitioner (GP), hospital and social services, housing, police and probation is paramount. Clearly, the better a patient is known, the more likely the accuracy of the risk assessment. If in doubt about the safety of continued community care of an individual prone to violence, admission should be considered.

The Royal College of Psychiatrists (1998) has produced clinical practice guidelines for the management of imminent violence. These cover ward design and organization, the need for adequate space, comfort and privacy, the anticipation and prevention of violence, including by fostering open communication with patients, anticipating risk and avoiding confrontation in a crisis, and training for staff to recognize warning signs of violence and to self-monitor verbal and non-verbal behaviour, and the appropriate use of medication. However, the guidelines acknowledge the lack of funding available for training, the shortage of qualified staff, and the levels of stress currently reported among those who work in the mental health field and deal with violence.

CONCLUSION

In summary, aim to determine how serious the risk of violence is, i.e. what are the nature and the magnitude of the risk? Is it specific or general, conditional or unconditional, immediate, long-term or volatile? Have the person's or the situation's risk factors changed? Who might be at risk?

From such a risk assessment, a risk-management plan should be developed to modify the risk factors and specify response triggers. This should, ideally, be agreed with the individual. Is there a need for more frequent follow-up appointments, an urgent CPA meeting or admission to hospital, detention under the Mental Health Act, physical security, observation and/or medication? If the optimum plan cannot be undertaken, then reasons for this should be documented and a back-up plan specified.

Risk assessments and risk-management plans should be communicated to others on a 'need-to-know' basis. On occasions, patient confidentiality will have to be breached if there is immediate grave danger to others. The police often can do little, unless there has been a specific threat to an individual, whereupon they may warn or charge the subject. Very careful consideration needs to be given before informing potential victims to avoid their unnecessary anxiety. Their safety is often best ensured by management of those who present the risk.

REFERENCES

Bennett, D (1996). Homicide, inquiries and scapegoating. *Psychiatric Bulletin* **20**, 298–300.

Boer, DP, Hart, SD, Kropp, PR, Webster, CD (1997). *Manual for the Sexual Violence Risk. Vol. 20: Professional Guidelines for Assessing Risk of Sexual Violence.* Vancouver: British Columbia Institute on Family Violence.

Department of Health (1990). *Health Circular: HC (90)23/LASSL(90)11 (The Care Programme Approach).* London: HMSO.

Farrington, DP (1995). The Twelfth Jack Tizard Memorial Lecture: the development of offending and antisocial behaviour from childhood: Key findings from the Cambridge Study in Delinquent Development. *Journal of Child Psychology and Psychiatry and Allied Disciplines* **36**, 929–64.

Hanson, RK, Thornton, D (1999). *Static 99: Improving Actuarial Risk Assessments for Sex Offenders. User Report 99-02.* Ottawa: Department of the Solicitor General of Canada.

Hanson, RK, Thornton, D (2000). Improving risk assessments for sex offenders: a comparison of three actuarial scales. *Law and Human Behaviour* **24**, 119–36.

Hare, RD (1991). *Manual for the Hare Psychopathy Checklist: Revised.* Toronto: Multi-Health Systems.

Hare, RD (2003). *Manual for the Hare Psychopathy Checklist: Revised (PCL-R™)*, 2nd edn. Toronto: Multi-Health Systems.

Harris, GT, Rice, ME, Quinsey, VL (1993). Violent recidivism of mentally disordered offenders: the development of a statistical prediction instrument. *Criminal Justice and Behaviour* **20**, 315-35.

Hart, SD, Cox, DN, Hare, RD (1995). *The Hare Psychopathy Checklist: Revised Screening Version (PCL-SV).* Toronto: Multi-Health Systems.

Humphreys, MS, Martin, S, Johnstone, EC, Macmillan, JF, Taylor, P (1992). Dangerous behaviour preceding first admission for schizophrenia. *British Journal of Psychiatry* **161**, 501–5.

Kropp, PR, Hart, SD, Webster, CW, Eaves, D (1995). *Manual for the Spousal Assault Risk Assessment Guide*, 2nd edn. Vancouver: British Columbia Institute on Family Violence.

Lidz, CW, Mulvey, EP, Gardner, W (1993). The accuracy of predictions of violence to others. *Journal of the American Medical Association* **269**, 1007–11.

Link, BG, Stueve, A (1994). Psychotic symptoms and violent/illegal behaviour of mental patients compared to community controls. In: Monahan, J, Steadman, J (eds). *Violence in Mental Disorder: Developments in Risk Assessment*. Chicago: University of Chicago Press, pp. 137–160.

Monaham, J, Steadman, HJ, Applebaum, PS, et al. (2000). Developing a clinically useful actuarial tool for assessing violence risk. *British Journal of Psychiatry* **176**, 312–20.

NHS Management Executive (1994a). *Introduction of Supervision Registers for Mentally Ill People from 1 April 1994: Health Service Guidelines HSG, (94)5*. London: Department of Health.

NHS Management Executive (1994b) *Guidance on the Discharge of Mentally Disordered People and Their Continuing Care in the Community: Health Service Guidelines HSG, (94)27*. London: Department of Health.

Quinsey, VL, Rice, ME, Harris, GT (1995). Actuarial prediction of sexual recidivism. *Journal of Interpersonal Violence* **10**, 85–105.

Quinsey, VL, Harris, GT, Rice, ME, Cormier, CA (1998). *Violent Offenders: Appraising and Managing Risk*. Washington, DC: American Psychological Association.

Ritchie, J, Dick, D, Lingham, R (1994). *Report of the Inquiry into the Care and Treatment of Christopher Clunis*. London: HMSO.

Royal College of Psychiatrists Special Working Party on Clinical Assessment and Management of Risk (1996). *Assessment and Clinical Management of Risk of Harm to Other People. Council Report CR53*. London: Royal College of Psychiatrists.

Royal College of Psychiatrists (1998). *Management of Imminent Violence. Clinical Practice Guidelines: Quick Reference Guide*. London: Royal College of Psychiatrists.

Steadman, HJ, Mulvey, EP, Monahan, J, Robbins PC, Appelbaum PS, Grisso T, et al. (1998). Violence by people discharged from acute psychiatric in-patient facilities and others in the same neighbourhoods. *Archives of General Psychiatry* **55**, 393–401.

Steadman, HJ, Silver, E, Monahan, J, Appelbaum, PS, Robbins, PC, Mulvey, EP, et al. (2000). Classification tree approach to the development of actuarial violence risk assessment tools. *Law and Human Behaviour* **24**, 83–100.

Swanson, JW, Holzer, CE, 3rd, Ganju, VK, Jono, RT (1990). Violence and psychiatric disorder in the community: evidence from epidemiologic catchment area survey. *Hospital and Community Psychiatry* **41**, 761–70.

Taylor, PJ (1993). Schizophrenia and crime: distinctive patterns in association. In: Hodgins, S (ed.). *Crime and Mental Disorder*. Beverly Hills, CA: Sage, pp. 63–85.

Taylor, PJ, Gunn, J (1999). Homicides by people with mental illness: myth and reality. *British Journal of Psychiatry* **174**, 9–14.

Webster, CD, Douglas, KS, Eaves, D, Hart, SD (1997). *HCR-20: Assessing Risk for Violence, Version 2*. Vancouver: Simon Fraser University Mental Health, Law and Policy Institute.

Wong, S, Gordon, A (2000). *Violence Risk Scale (VRS)*. Saskatchewan: Department of Psychology and Research. Regional Psychiatric Centre: Solicitor General of Canada.

16

Suicidal patients

Suicide is defined in the Oxford English Dictionary as the 'intentional killing of oneself' and in Webster's Third New International Dictionary (1968) as 'the act or an instance of taking one's own life by a person of years of discretion and of sound mind: one that commits or attempts self-murder'. Its practical and emotional consequences are felt by family and friends particularly but also colleagues, professionals and all who were involved closely with the deceased.

EPIDEMIOLOGY

Suicide is an important public-health issue. Each year, between 4000 and 6000 people kill themselves, and it is sometimes said that one person takes their own life every two hours in England. Approximately 2000 people die from asthma and a further 2000 from cervical cancer over a similar period.

Older men used to have the highest suicide death rate, but they now appear to be eclipsed by younger men. Suicide and accidents are the commonest cause of death in men under 35 years of age.

Risk factors for successful completion of suicide include male sex, living alone, mental illness, unemployment, substance misuse and previous self-harm.

The suicide rate varies from country to country, and the rate also varies in different cultures and religions. Hungary is the country with the highest number of completed suicides worldwide. Certain occupations appear to have a higher risk of completed suicide, including farming, veterinary science, pharmacy, medicine and social work; this may be because access to lethal means of suicide, such as guns, weedkillers and drugs, is relatively easy. In the case of farmers and vets, the philosophy also exists that an ailing animal should be put out of its misery, which may influence how they feel about humans.

Methods of suicide seem to depend upon the availability of an appropriate lethal way of killing oneself. The intended suicide victim needs to have private access to a suitable place, such as a bridge over a river, the roof of a tall building, or a railway line. Women tend to use less violent methods compared with men, such as overdose of medication or attaching a hosepipe to a car exhaust pipe.

HISTORY OF SUICIDE ATTITUDES AND LEGISLATION

The morality of suicide has provoked many strong emotions over the centuries. Aristotle and Plato felt that it was 'an offence against all the gods of all the state'.

In common law, suicide was seen as a form of felonious homicide that offended both God and the king. It offended God because the person in question rushed into His presence when 'uncalled for' and offended the king because he 'hath interest in the preservation of all his subjects'. A person who completed suicide successfully had his or her estate seized; the body was placed at the crossroads of two highways and a stake driven through it. In France, the body was hung, drawn and quartered. This attitude prevailed until 1823, when it was relaxed a little, but the body still could not be buried in consecrated ground.

However, there have always been conflicting feelings about suicide. The Roman Stoics condoned suicide and felt that 'it was a lawful and rational exercise of individual freedom and even wise in the cases of old age'.

As it was difficult to prosecute people who had killed themselves and were dead, the law concentrated on prosecuting people who attempted suicide. This continued until the **Suicide Act 1961** became law.

The Suicide Act 1961

Section 1 of the Suicide Act 1961 stated that attempting suicide was no longer to be considered a crime. The attitude of society in general had ameliorated to suicide before this legislation, but suicide still remained a social stigma.

Section 2(1) states that anyone who aids, abets, counsels or procures the suicide of another, or an attempt by another, to commit suicide is liable upon conviction on indictment to imprisonment for a term not exceeding 14 years.

Case law

Case law illustrating some of the above points was *AG* v. *Able* (1984) 1 ALL ER 277. In this case, a voluntary euthanasia committee published a booklet, *A Guide to Self Deliverance*, setting out in detail methods of committing suicide with an expressed aim of helping to overcome a fear of dying and to decrease the number of failed attempts. The Attorney General took the view that this constituted an offence under Section 2(1) of the Suicide Act 1961. Wolf J in his deliberations concluded that he did consider that the distribution of the booklet could be an offence. However, before it can be established that an offence has been committed, it must be proved that the alleged offender had the necessary intent. The offender needed to intend that the booklet be used by someone contemplating suicide and that the person should be assisted by the book's contents; also, for the offence to be proven, it was necessary to prove that the person was encouraged or assisted by reading the booklet to take or attempt to take his or her own life.

Physician-assisted suicide

This occurs when a person is assisted by a doctor to commit suicide. It usually occurs in the setting of a painful terminal illness such as cancer or a degenerative neurological disease. It contravenes Section 2(1) of the Suicide Act 1961.

It has often been argued that the law relating to doctor-assisted suicide should be changed, since patients are denied control over their own deaths. Throughout the years, there has been media attention on a number of occasions concerning this topic. In 1990, Jack Kevorkian, a retired pathologist, enabled a woman in the early stages of Alzheimer's disease to kill herself; he received unanimous condemnation. In the case of *Rodriquez v. British Columbia* (A-G) (1993) 82 BCLR (2d) 273 (Can Sc), a patient suffering from amyotrophic lateral sclerosis wished to avoid choking to death. She wanted to have an intravenous line installed, which contained a substance that she would choose to use when she decided to end her life. Her application and appeal were dismissed.

Another important case was that of *Secretary of State for the Home Department* v. *Robb* (1995) 1 ALL ER 677. In 1994, a respondent prisoner who had been diagnosed as suffering from a personality disorder went on hunger strike. He was of sound mind and understood the situation. The Home Secretary sought a declaration that the Home Office, prison officials, physicians and nurses might lawfully observe and abide by the respondent's wishes. Since the prisoner was refusing treatment, it could be construed that he was committing suicide, and the doctors were concerned that they could be found guilty of an offence under Section 2(1) of the Suicide Act 1961. Thorpe J deliberated and said that if a man refused, however unreasonably, to accept treatment and died, then he had not committed suicide. The doctors, therefore, were not guilty of aiding and abetting suicide and it would be lawful not to force-feed the respondent.

The only other previous similar case was a suffragette who had been force-fed and sought damages against the Home Secretary. At that time, suicide was a criminal act and the people attending her could have been guilty of a crime. The woman was not successful in her claim, and the verdict was qualified by a statement that it was a time of 'dramatic conflict'.

In some other countries, such as the Netherlands, physician-assisted suicide is illegal. Article 294 of the Dutch Supreme Court states: 'A person who intentionally incites another to commit suicide, assists in the suicide of another or procures for that person the means to commit suicide is liable to a term of imprisonment of not more than three years where the suicide ensues.' However, the Dutch Supreme Court has recognized that a doctor who assists in suicide under certain circumstances is not guilty of an offence under the Dutch Criminal Code. He or she has the defence of 'necessity' but must conform to all the regulations. A Dutch psychiatrist, Dr Chabot, in June 1994 was the first to assist the suicide of a woman, Helly Boscher, for a psychological reason, namely depression. Although he had asked others for a second opinion, he had nothing in writing and was found guilty under Article 294, but he did not receive any sentence.

In 1994, the Select Committee's Report stated: 'The Government can see no basis for permitting assisted suicide. Such a change would be open to abuse and put the lives of the weak and vulnerable at risk.'

'Slippery slope'

There is fear that physician-assisted suicide could lead to mistrust and abuse and damage the relationship that hopefully exists between patients and doctors. Furthermore, a physician could agree to help a patient to commit suicide when the patient is clinically depressed and all other avenues, such as pain relief and family feelings, have not been explored, and thus it may be practised to an increasing degree. The Law Reform Commission suggests that in order to protect life and those who are vulnerable in society, a prohibition without exception on assisted suicide is the best approach. When there have been attempts to fine-tune things, such as in the Netherlands, it has been unsatisfactory and has supported the 'slippery-slope' theory.

The Human Rights Act 1998

There have been arguments that the above attitude was not compatible with the Human Rights Act 1998. The English courts do not have the power to disapply the Suicide Act 1961, even if it were found to be incompatible with the Human Rights Act 1998.

An English woman who was dying of motor neurone disease and wished to avoid a frightening and undignified death from choking applied for permission for her husband to be able to help her die without being charged under the Suicide Act 1961. Her application was dismissed, as was her appeal. She then went to the European Court of Human Rights – *Pretty (R on the app of)* v. *DPP and SS* – on the grounds that it was against her human rights to be denied a dignified death. This was also dismissed, and it was stated that there was no power to ensure that her husband was not prosecuted.

Article 2.1 states that everyone's life shall be protected by law. No one shall be deprived intentionally of his or her life, except in the execution of a sentence of court following a crime for which the penalty is provided by law. Article 3 also protects the right to live with as much dignity as can be afforded until life reaches its natural end.

Hopes had been pinned on Article 8, which states that everyone has the right to respect for private and family life without interference by a public authority. This can occur only in accordance with the law and in the interests of national security.

It was concluded that the right to life did not include the right to die at a time and manner of one's choice. This was not compatible with the Convention, it having legitimate aims of upholding the value of life and protecting vulnerable people.

PALLIATIVE CARE

Palliative care is medical care of people who are terminally ill. It has as part of its philosophy the administration of drugs designed for pain control in dosages that may hasten the death of the patient. The doctor knows this but is using the drugs with the intent not of causing death but of easing pain.

The distinction, then, between palliative care and assisted suicide or euthanasia is that the former is to ease pain and the latter is to cause death. The term 'double-effect' has been used to describe medication being used for pain relief also speeding up death. It would be unfortunate if people were to suffer because of concerns about administering drugs that might speed up death. However, in some cases, there is a possibility that someone will commit euthanasia or assist suicide under the guise of palliative care and will not be caught because of the difficulty of getting proof.

NATIONAL CONFIDENTIAL ENQUIRY INTO PATIENT OUTCOME AND DEATH (NCEPOD)

The Health of the Nation White Paper published in 1992 stated that the government had set a target for reducing the overall suicide rate by at least 15 per cent and the suicide rate of severely mentally ill people by 33 per cent by the year 2000.

The Department of Health also established a Confidential Enquiry into Homicides and Suicides by Mentally Ill People. The purpose was to find out avoidable causes of death and set standards for best practice. This was to be done by examining by questionnaire the circumstances surrounding any death that occurred. The Confidential Enquiry's terms of reference included looking at the circumstances leading up to and surrounding the suicides of people discharged by specialist psychiatric services. The first report looked at 240 suicides; 154 of these were outpatients and 53 were inpatients.

The most common event was the breakdown of marriage or partnership; two-thirds of the people were living on their own. Social and employment problems were common. The most common psychiatric diagnoses were schizophrenia and personality disorder. Previous self-harm was reported in more than half of the cases, and aggression was reported in 32 per cent.

The conclusions reached by the group emphasized marital breakdown, social isolation, bereavement, lack of employment, low social-work input and poor care planning as factors. The report supposes that the hopelessness about the future on the patient's side against a professional's perception of relevant treatment and supervision as well as surprise at the act require more attention to be given to the patient's view about whether his or her treatment is relevant to the situation.

RISK ASSESSMENT OF SUICIDE

The Blueglass and Horton six-item scale is a suicide predictor and lists the following:

- alcohol misuse
- previous diagnosis of personality disorder
- previous inpatient treatment
- previous outpatient treatment
- previous suicide attempt leading to hospital admission
- not living with a relative.

This suicide scale is used by allocating points for any of the six items indicated above that are present. Persons with several of the problems listed in the scale have a greater risk of completing suicide than someone who has none of the above.

Other scales include the Beck Suicide Intent Scale and the Tuckman and Youngman Scale.

A weakness of these scales is that they concentrate on things that are hopeless and that cannot be helped; they do not look at anything positive. It may be the loss of a positive object that will precipitate suicide.

A clinical interview is also very useful for assessing risk of suicide and should not be overlooked because of the medicolegal requirement for tick-box risk assessments.

NATIONAL SUICIDE PREVENTION STRATEGY FOR ENGLAND

Consultation document

The consultation document was published in April 2002 and sets out the components of the National Suicide Prevention Strategy. It is hoped that this evolving document will implement the reduction in suicide set in *Our Healthier Nation* of one-fifth by the year 2010. The document sets out six goals for suicide prevention:

- To reduce the availability and lethality of suicide methods.
- To reduce risk among high-risk groups.
- To promote mental wellbeing in the wider population.
- To improve the reporting of suicidal behaviour in the media.
- To promote research on suicide prevention.
- To improve the monitoring of progress towards the target set out in *Our Healthier Nation*.

The document looks at each goal and breaks it down before deciding upon a strategy for each particular goal. An example of this is Objective 2.4, which is to reduce the number of deaths of prisoners, a high-risk group, by 20 per cent. Fourteen actions have already been taken, and a further two are for consultation.

The document also looks at death by hanging and medication and considers ways of improving the situation.

National Service Framework for Mental Health

This is a minimum set of standards for promoting mental health and care for all. There are similar standards for diabetes and paediatrics. Standard 7 – Preventing Suicide looks at the epidemiology of suicide and then focuses on service models and good practice, with emphasis on care-management and operational issues.

CONCLUSION

Suicide is a complex issue that gives rise to strong feelings and causes acute distress. It is influenced by religious and cultural aspects of life, and there is a large variation from country to country. Society has a strong sense of preservation of life and tries to reduce the number of people killing themselves, but there has always been a significant number of people for whom suicide is very seductive.

REFERENCE

Department of Health (1999). Saving Lives: Our Healthier Nation (OHN) White Paper. London: The Stationery Office.

17

Children's mental health law

INTRODUCTION

Children and young people in the UK are subject to a potentially confusing combination of legislation according to their stage of development, their maturity, and how they present. Their degree of autonomy and independent participation in the process also vary with the above and other factors. The main legislation in addition to the Mental Health Act 1983 is the Children Act 1989 and also common law/case law.

Mental health professionals may be asked or required to give evidence in civil or criminal proceedings where the child or adolescent is a witness, alleged victim, alleged perpetrator or simply offspring or relative of another individual involved in proceedings. Evidence may relate to the child or adolescent or some aspect of behaviour of an adult towards that child or adolescent (most notably parenting) (Brophy 2001).

MENTAL HEALTH ACT 1983

The Mental Health Act 1983 in its principal provisions does not have any age specifications. The exception in the Act is the guardianship order (Section 37). It is not intended that this be used in respect of children (legally, any person under the age of 18 years is a child.) However, specifically, patients may be received into guardianship only if they have reached the age of 16 years. There are three specific powers invested in the guardian (to require the patient to live at a particular place, to require the patient to attend specific places at specific times, and to require access to the patient by people specified by the guardian). In a child, these can be carried out by a person with 'parental responsibility' (see later) or under specific provisions of the Children Act.

The Mental Health (Patients in the Community) Act 1995 similarly excludes children under the age of 16 years from the provision of a supervised discharge order.

The explanatory Memorandum to the Mental Health Act (Department of Health 1998) contains a few brief references regarding children and young people, but this was expanded and elaborated in the Code of Practice (Department of Health 1999, Chapter 31).

The Code of Practice clarifies further that, in addition to the age limit on guardianship, a patient must have attained the age of 16 years to be subject to aftercare under supervision (Section 25a).

The legal requirements to provide information are also elaborated on in the Code of Practice. It is stated that all professionals, local social services authorities, educational authorities and Trusts should ensure that the necessary information (including the Code of Practice, the Act, the Children Act and volumes 1,4 6 and 7 of Children Act guidance) is available to those responsible for the care of children. This also applies to those young people who have sufficient maturity and understanding to participate more fully in the process.

Consideration of whether to use the Mental Health Act or the Children Act in circumstances where it is thought necessary to require residence or to insist on a particular course of treatment is not always straightforward. In the first instance, it is important to establish the primary purpose of using the law. The Mental Health Act, the Children Act and associated literature affirm repeatedly that the law should be used only where it would be unsafe not to do so. It must be shown that the child's or young person's health or welfare would be better served by using the law than by not doing so. In other words, non-statutory action is always preferred, all other things being equal.

If a child or young person is thought to be suffering from a serious mental illness, then the Mental Health Act should be used. Conversely, serious behaviour disturbance, in the absence of mental illness, may be dealt with better with a secure accommodation order or a Section 8 order under the Children Act (see later). One possible complication is that 'conduct disorder' is classified in both the fourth edition of the *Diagnostic and Statistical Manual of Mental Disorders* (DSM-IV-TR) (American Psychiatric Association 2000) and the tenth edition of the *International Classification of Diseases* (ICD-10) (World Health Organization 1992) as a 'disorder'. This, it may be argued, makes the case of a young person with serious behaviour problems suitable for use of the Mental Health Act. In practice, this does not happen at present. Whether forthcoming revisions of the Mental Health Act, particularly regarding 'personality disorder', will confuse the picture further remains to be seen.

At the time of writing, there is a strong push by the UK government to encourage a close working relationship between the various agencies so that there is usually, in non-emergency cases, some sort of joint panel considering funding of placement and the sharing of cost according to social care, health or educational need. This must be distinguished from the decision about legal action. Individual approved officers (social workers and doctors) make decisions about the use of the Mental Health Act, whereas the use of the Children Act is an agency decision by social services in conjunction with other statutory authorities. In the Children Act, the power is the function of the local authority rather than individual agents of that authority.

The Mental Health Act Code of Practice states that staff considering the above should:

(a) be aware of the relevant statutory provisions and have easy access to competent legal advice;

(b) keep in mind the importance of ensuring the child's care is managed with clarity, consistency and within a recognisable framework; and

(c) attempt to select the option that reflects the predominant needs to the child at that time whether that be to provide specific mental health care and treatment or to achieve a measure of safety and protection. Either way the least restrictive option consistent with the care and treatment objectives for the child should be sought.

Guiding principles

Also in the Code of Practice, additional considerations for children and young people are:

- *Having regard to their age and understanding,* they should be kept as fully informed as possible about their care and treatment and their views and wishes found out and taken into account. Particular mention is made of having regard to the impact of the children's wishes on their parents and/or others with parental responsibility. (In some places, this was thought to indicate that the court and others must always agree with the child, but it is clear that this is not what is intended. Subsequent judgments have confirmed this. Conversely, the child's view will carry more weight in proceedings, with increasing age and maturity; see later section on consent.)
- The assumption is that the least restrictive course is taken and, in particular, giving least possible segregation from family, friends, community and school.
- All children and young people in hospital should receive appropriate education (The Education of Sick Children, DfEE circular 12/94, DH circulars LAC(94)10 and HSG(94)24, May 1994).

It will also be important for professionals to consider:

- who has 'parental responsibility' for the child or young person (see later);
- if the parents are separated, whether there is a residence order and whether both parents should be contacted?
- the child's emotional maturity, intellectual capacity and mental state, with respect to consent;
- where the person with parental responsibility has refused consent to treatment, the soundness of the reasons and the grounds on which they refuse;
- whether the child's needs could be met elsewhere (social services, education placements) and whether all the possibilities have been considered.

Informal admission

In paragraphs 31.6–31.9 of the Code of Practice, the rather complicated issues dealing with consent are explained for the first time. This is elaborated further in paragraphs 31.10–31.16 (consent to medical treatment).

  A key issue is that of Gillick competency. This derives from a court decision in the case of *Gillick* v. *West Norfolk and Wisbech Area Health Authority and another* (1986) AC112. This court case was concerned with whether a young person under the age of 16 years could consent to medical treatment with contraceptives without their parents' permission or knowledge. The judgment was that where a doctor concludes that such a child under the age of 16 years has the capacity to make such a decision for him- or herself (i.e. he or she is of sufficient intelligence and understanding to make that decision), then the child can legally consent. The General Medical Council (GMC) in respect of doctors makes it clear that in addition it is good practice that, as far as possible, efforts should be made to persuade a young person that the involvement of the parents or a person with parental responsibility is advisable. A further case in the Court of Appeal (*Re R* (1992) 1 FLR 190) stated that Gillick competence is a developmental concept and, as such, will not be lost or acquired on a day-to-day or week-to-week basis. Where there is mental disability that must also be taken into account, particularly where there is a possibility of the disability fluctuating in its effect, Gillick competency has been extended beyond the original issue (prescription of contraception) to other areas where an adult might give consent for a child. The Code of Practice makes it clear that included in this is consent to informal admission to hospital (Paragraph 31.6). It is expected that the views of parents or those with parental responsibility would be checked. However, if a Gillick competent child is willing to be admitted, then the parents' views should be taken into account, but the view of the child would ordinarily prevail. However, the converse is not currently the case. In *Re W* (1992) 4 All ER 627 (a case regarding the treatment of a young person with anorexia nervosa), it was stated that the refusal of a Gillick competent child to be treated medically can be overridden by the court or by his or her parents. At the time of writing, the legality of this under the Human Rights Act 1998 has not been tested.

For 16- and 17-year-olds, there is no question as to whether they can consent to informal admission to hospital (and to medical treatment), providing they are of 'sound mind'. However, if the person is incapable of expressing his or her own wishes, then the parents' consent should be sought, or consideration may need to be given to whether a patient should be detained under the Mental Health Act. The decision about which course to take will be influenced by clinical considerations, such as the importance of maintaining collaboration with all parties. Statutory access to appeals etc. may mean that use of the Mental Health Act is preferred.

The court may need to be involved where the child is under the age of 16 years or is not Gillick competent but treatment decisions need to be made and the person with parental responsibility cannot be identified or is incapacitated, or it is apparent that the person with parental responsibility may not be acting in the best interests of the child in making treatment decisions on behalf of the child. Despite the fact that courts and those with parental responsibility may override a child's refusal to be treated, it is stated that this refusal is 'a very important consideration in making clinical judgements … its importance increases with the age and maturity of the child' (Code of Practice Paragraph 13.13).

Further issues dealing with involvement with medical services are considered in the Children Act (see later). Sixteen- and 17-year-olds can normally consent to any surgical, medical or dental treatment, despite officially being 'minors' (Family Law Reform Act 1987). Where a 16- or 17-year-old is incapable, then the parents or another person with parental responsibility can give consent on the patient's behalf and also can override the patient's refusal to consent (although, as before, this is only if the *Re W* decision is binding and applied, having not been overridden by the Human Rights Act.)

In an emergency situation, a doctor may give treatment if delay would be dangerous. The Code of Practice states that it would be good practice in this situation to attempt to obtain the consent of parents or those with parental responsibility.

THE CHILDREN ACT 1989

The Children Act 1989, which was implemented in October 1991, was a major piece of legislation that brought together much of the law relating to children in England and Wales and introduced a number of new concepts together with a fundamental shift to make the child's interest central to consideration rather than the rights of the various adults involved. The concept of the 'family' and the need to reinforce the autonomy of this unit through the exercise of parental responsibility is a core feature. The Act also brings together private law (e.g. divorces) and public law (e.g. care proceedings) in a way that addresses the needs of the child.

Principles of the Act

- The *child's welfare is paramount* (this has been extended to cover consent and has also been included as a principle within UK GMC advice to doctors about appropriate practice).
- The concept of *parental responsibility* (see below) was introduced to replace 'parental rights'.
- The Act *allows children to be parties to proceedings* in their own right, separate from their parents.
- *Identification of children in need* and safeguarding and promoting their welfare are identified explicitly as duties for local authorities in partnership with others (especially parents).
- The Act and its guidance include duties and powers for local authorities to provide certain services for children and families.
- The *welfare checklist* was introduced into courts as a mandatory part of the decision-making process (see Table 17.1).
- The *no-order principle* directs courts and others involved in proceedings to make sure that any order made is better for the child than making no order at all.
- There is an explicit assumption that delay in deciding questions concerning children is prejudicial to their welfare and that in all proceedings this will be minimized.

Structure of the Act

The Act is arranged in 12 parts and 15 schedules (see Table 17.2). In this chapter, only those parts of the Children Act with which Mental Health workers are more

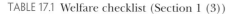

TABLE 17.1 Welfare checklist (Section 1 (3))

Used in opposed applications for Section 8 orders and in care proceedings. Having determined the ascertainable wishes and feelings of the child (considered in the light of his or her age and understanding), it is incumbent on the Court to decide in the best interests of the child. This does not always concord with the child's wishes, but it will vary according to the age and development. The court must consider the following:

Physical, emotional and educational needs of the child

Likely effect on the child of any change in circumstances

Age, sex, background and any characteristics that the court considers relevant to the child

Any harm that the child has suffered or is at risk of suffering

The capability of each of the child's parents and the other person in relation to the child if the court considers the question to be relevant to meeting the child's needs

The range of powers available to the court in the proceedings in question

TABLE 17.2 Parts of the Children Act 1989

Part	Title	Description
1	Introductory	Welfare of children is paramount; concept of parental responsibility introduced
2	Orders in respect of children and family proceedings	(Replacing previous concepts of custody, care, control and access); includes Section 8 orders
3	Local Authority support for children and families	Provision for accommodation by local authorities; concept of 'looked-after children' introduced to replace 'in care'
4	Care and supervision	'Threshold criteria' introduced for care orders
5	Protection of children	Introduced the Child Assessment Order and Emergency Protection Order with duties to investigate
6	Community homes	
7	Voluntary homes and voluntary organizations	
8	Registered children's homes	
9	Private arrangements for fostering children	
10	Child-minding and day care for young children	
11	The Secretary of State supervisory functions and responsibilities	
12	Miscellaneous and general	

likely to be involved are considered (parts 1–5). The reader is directed to the Children Act itself or one of the several guides available (e.g. Clarke Hall and Morrison 1990, Mitchels and Prince 1992) for details of the other sections and their implementation.

Parental responsibility

Parental responsibility is defined as 'all the rights, duties, powers, responsibilities and authority which by law the parent of a child has in relation to the child and his property'. Parental responsibility is accorded automatically to the child's father and mother if they are married to each other at or after the child's birth. If the parents are unmarried, then the mother has parental responsibility but the father does not unless he acquires it. The father can acquire parental responsibility by application to the court; by making a Parental Responsibility Agreement between the father and mother; by being appointed as a guardian by the court, the mother or another guardian; or, since December 2003, by being registered as the child's father. Guardians or others appointed by the court or a parent can acquire parental responsibility (Section 5). Just because another person acquires parental responsibility does not negate the responsibility of those already having parental responsibility. Parental responsibility can be lost only by adoption (or freeing for adoption).

Child welfare

Child welfare is the paramount consideration of the court. This includes establishing a timetable and giving directions for the appropriate handling of a case to minimize delay. Also, Section 1(5) establishes the 'no-order principle', i.e. a specific reason for establishing an order needs to be established.

Children in need

Health authority workers or workers in other agencies can be involved under Section 27 of the Act in which local authorities are allowed to request the help of other authorities or people in relation to specified actions. The authorities are directed to comply with requests if this is compatible with their own statutory duties and obligations and does not unduly prejudice the discharge of any of their functions (clearly, this gives considerable scope!). The document *Working Together Under the Children Act 1989* (Department of Health 1991) enlarges on this principle.

The emphasis on promoting the welfare of children in need is set out in detail in Part 3 of the Act. This replaced the rather negative previous duty of the local authority to provide services that prevented children being taken into care. The other side of the coin, however, is the provision of child-protection services in conjunction with other agencies to investigate and manage situations where there is evidence of abuse. Even where there is evidence of significant harm, the following principles still apply:

■ minimal intrusion;

- voluntary arrangements if possible;
- no order if this would be better for the child;
- child returned to the family wherever possible, if this is in the child's interests,

Partnership

The Children Act makes it clear that partnership is a key component of any intervention affecting a child. The partnership is between services and those with parental responsibility and between all the services working with a child of the family. Thus, even if a child is 'in care' – i.e. social care services have parental responsibility for the child or the child is 'looked after' by social care services – this does not obviate the necessity to work with those others who have parental responsibility (most notably the parents). This is limited if the child is in care by Section 33 (iii), which gives the local authority the power to determine the degree to which a parent or guardian can exercise their parental responsibility, if this is in the interest of the child's welfare.

The concept of partnership also acknowledges that intervention by outside agencies in a child's relationship with his or her carers may itself be inadvertently damaging or prejudicial to the child's welfare. For example:

- attendance of the child at court (American Academy of Pediatrics 1999);
- multiple and repeated interviewing (Spencer and Flin 1993);
- making decisions that minimize the risk of future legal action against the agency;
- multiple placements (ignoring the importance of the child's needs for a healthy attachment).

Court proceedings

Rather than designating a specific court in which a particular order is considered or power is held, the Children Act introduced a more flexible system that allowed the level of court (its expertise in the law) to be matched to the level of complexity of the case. The usual system of appeals to higher courts remains. The basic court is a Magistrate's Court that is designated a 'family proceedings court', with magistrates who receive special training to be on the 'family panel'. Both private and public law cases may be heard at these courts.

At the next level of County Courts, some are designated 'family hearing centres' to hear private law cases. A smaller number are designated 'care centres' and hear public law applications. A 'family judge' sits at either of these centres. 'Designated family' or 'nominated' judges may sit at care centres to hear either public or private applications. 'Circuit family' judges sit at family hearing centres to hear only private law applications.

Above the County Courts is the Family Division of the High Court.

These courts all have access to the full range of powers and orders under the Children Act, i.e. there is *concurrent jurisdiction*.

The court is required, in a *directions hearing*, to set a timetable and other arrangements for the preparation of the case so that a final hearing can go ahead.

At this stage, the question of expert assessments and evidence is considered and arranged, if necessary. The relative lack of availability of professionals to act as expert witnesses has meant that initial expectations of hearings occurring within 3 months at most have not been met (Brophy 2001).

The guardian *ad litem*

The guardian *ad litem* (GAL) is an officer appointed by the court in public law applications to safeguard the interests of the child. The GAL will appoint lawyers on behalf of the child, and on behalf of the court, and will consider all aspects of the child's experience and likely experience, including the child's experience of statutory services. The GAL has full access to the files of social care services. They will not only interview and report on the wishes and viewpoint of the child but also investigate the views of all others that impinge or may in future affect the child (e.g. prospective foster parents). The GAL will advise the court on the child's level of understanding (e.g. for purposes of consent to medical examination). They may advise the court or may themselves instruct expert witnesses. Latterly, the wish to minimize the number of examinations of the child has made it more likely that the court or GAL instructs a single expert or team. Also, where there is more than one expert in a case, they can be instructed to meet with each other in order to come to a consensus or, at the least, identify all the areas on which they agree.

GALs usually come from a senior social work, probation or court welfare background. (The equivalent in private law applications is the court welfare officer.) In the early days of the Children Act, GALs and court welfare officers were employed differently (the GAL was part of the Guardian ad litem and Reporting Officers Service under the aegis of the local authority). However, since spring 2001, both sets of court officers comprise the Children and Families Courts Advice and Support Service (CAFCASS.)

Orders under the Children Act

See Table 17.3.

Public law orders

A care or supervision order may be made only where the threshold criteria are satisfied (see Figure 17.1). However, the no-order principle must be satisfied.

Significant harm

'Significant harm' is a key legal issue in the child protection part of the Children Act 1989. In Section 31(2) of the Children Act, a court may make a care order or supervision order in respect to a particular child only if it is satisfied that:

- the child concerned is likely to suffer *significant harm; and*
- the harm or likelihood of harm is attributable to:
  - *the care* given, or likely to be given, to the child if the order were not

TABLE 17.3　Orders under the Children Act 1989

Order	Section
Public law orders	
Care order	31
Interim care order	38
Contact with children in care	34
Supervision order	31
Education supervision order	36
Interim supervision order	38
Child assessment order	43
Emergency protection order	44–45
Recovery order	50
Private law orders	
Residence order	8
Contact order	8
Specific issues order	8
Prohibited steps order	8
Family assistance order	16

made not being what it would be reasonable to expect a parent to give to a similar child; *or*
– the child being beyond parental control.

Section 31(9) defines 'harm' as ill-treatment or 'impairment of health or development', although they may coexist in an interactive or non-interactive manner.

'Ill treatment' includes sexual abuse and non-physical emotional abuse. Identification of the perpetrator(s) by the court is often necessary in order to sort out whether this or failure to prevent harm is part of parental care. The 'proof' is of a lower order (balance of probabilities) than in criminal proceedings, where the 'beyond reasonable doubt' principle applies.

'Health or development' refers to both mental and physical health; development is physical, intellectual, emotional or behavioural development.

Reference to a 'similar child' makes it clear that in an individual case, the presence or absence of extra difficulties will have a bearing on the expected parenting required to satisfy the court. It must be emphasized that the standard of parenting must be reasonable rather than best, otherwise a child could be removed because allegedly better foster arrangements are available.

'Likely to suffer' means that a one-off incident from which there are no long-term sequelae will not in itself satisfy the criteria. The likelihood of repetition (e.g. of parental depression or drug use) of a harmful event or set of harmful environmental circumstances will influence the court. 'Likely' is taken to mean more than a possibility but less than 'more likely than not', i.e. a possibility of about one in three.

SIGNIFICANT HARM CRITERIA

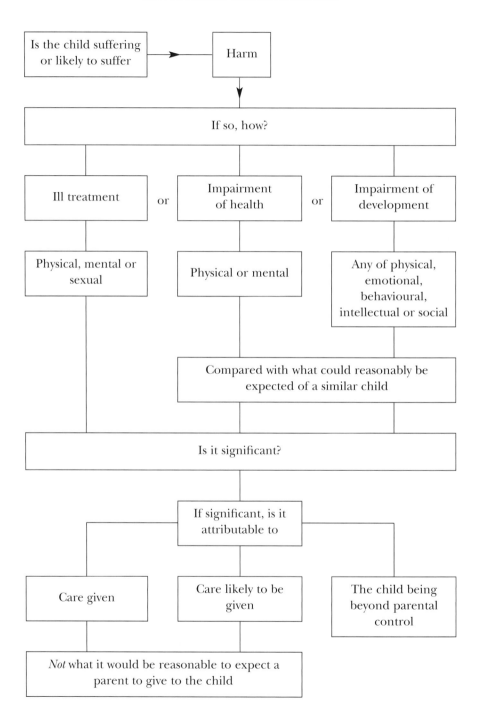

FIGURE 17.1 Diagram summarizing threshold criteria. (Reproduced with kind permission from Adcock, A, White, R (1998). *Significant Harm: Its Management and Outcome*, 2nd edn. London: Significant Publications, p. 4.)

After the threshold criteria are satisfied, the court considers the welfare checklist and the paramountcy of the child's welfare (Section 1(3)). An expert witness may be asked to express an opinion on the former to help guide the court. Even if all of the above are satisfied, the care or supervision order may not be made as the court is required to consider all possible interventions, including Section 8 orders. (As noted above, such orders may be made without threshold criteria being satisfied and without application from any of the parties involved.)

DEFINITIONS OF ABUSE

Significant harm may be considered as 'a compilation of significant events, both acute and longstanding, which interact with the child's ongoing development and interrupt, alter or impair physical and psychological development' (Bentovim 1991). Comprehensive social care assessment, as detailed in the *Framework for the Assessment of Children in Need and Their Families* (Department of Health 2000), is a systematic effort to tease out the factors contributing to the presenting predicament, their relative weights, their interactions and their possibilities for amelioration. In all the categories of abuse, inadequate care may comprise acts of commission and/or omission. In other words, inadequate or inappropriate parenting may fail to protect from abuse as well as commit acts of abuse.

Before a *care order* is made, the court is required to consider the arrangements made by the local authority regarding contact of specific people with a child and must invite the parties to the proceedings to comment on these (Section 34). It must be noted that Section 34 obviates the needs (and the ability under the Children Act) for the local authority to use a Section 8 contact order.

Supervision orders may include conditions and medical or psychiatric examination or treatment (subject to consent as below). A supervision order designates a 'supervisor' (usually the local authority), who is under a duty to:

- advise, assist and befriend the child;
- take steps 'as reasonably necessary' to carry out the order;
- consider applying for a variation or discharge if the order is no longer necessary or is not being complied with.

Directions about the actions and activities of the child and the 'responsible person' may be included in the order.

The *education supervision order* is used specifically for circumstances in which a child is not attending school.

In the period of time between application and decision regarding making an order, the court has a choice of:

- a Section 8 order (see private law orders, below)
- an interim care order
- an interim supervision order.

An *interim care order* may be made when a care-order application is adjourned or with directions to investigate a child's circumstances. The local authority must provide accommodation, maintain the child, and allow reasonable contact with those with parental responsibility. All of the following apply:

- welfare paramountcy
- delays likely to be prejudicial
- no-order presumption
- welfare checklist.

The interim care order is for eight weeks, with the option of extension up to 12 weeks. There is no limit to the number of the interim care orders, but the above principles must be borne in mind and the provision of a timetable for the proceedings is required.

The main differences between interim and full care and supervision orders are that (i) directions may be made in the former, and (ii) the durations of the orders are more restricted in interim orders.

One of the above temporary orders may be made only if the court is satisfied that there are *reasonable grounds* to believe that the threshold criteria (Section 31 (2)) are met. When a residence order is made, an interim supervision order is also made, unless the court is satisfied that the child will be protected without one.

Child protection orders

Child assessment order (Section 43)

A child assessment order under the Children Act may be applied for by the local authority or an authorized person. It lasts for seven days and may not be applied for again within the next six months without leave of the court. The court has to be satisfied that:

- the child is suffering, or is likely to suffer, significant harm;
- an assessment is required that would determine this;
- it is not possible to perform such as assessment without an order (and attempts to carry out an assessment without an order have failed).

The effect of the order is to require a child's carer or person with parental responsibility to produce a child at a particular time to the person (assessor) referred to in the order. In addition, an assessment in accordance with the order is authorized (not applicable where a child can give valid consent him- or herself).

This order is applicable where there are longstanding concerns rather than an emergency arising and will be preceded by a full social care assessment (Section 47). Keeping the child away from home is allowed but should be minimized and planned for.

Emergency protection order (sections 44 and 45)

The Children Act warns specifically that a child assessment order must not be made if the grounds for an emergency protection order are met. Anyone may apply for an emergency protection order. The grounds for an emergency protection order are as follows:

- the child will suffer significant harm if not removed from his or her current predicament;

- urgent access is required and is being unreasonably withheld;
- if the applicant is 'an authorized person', there is reasonable cause to suspect that the child is suffering significant harm;
- enquiries are being thwarted and emergency access is required.

The order requires any person who can produce the child to do so. The order may determine that a child is to be moved to accommodation supplied by the applicant or that removal, e.g. from hospital, is to be prevented. The applicant acquires parental responsibility under the order.

When the emergency protection order is in force, the court can make directions regarding contact and also regarding medical or psychiatric assessment, within the bounds of consent as mentioned previously.

A warrant may be issued by the court to a police constable to help any person carrying out the order (including using force), where refusal of access to the child is evident or is likely.

The emergency protection order lasts eight days, with possible extension to 15 days. Longer periods of time may be ordered when the emergency protection order ends on a public holiday or a Sunday. Discharge of the order must occur for as long as it is safe to do so.

Recovery order (Section 50)

This is an order that the court may make in cases of child abduction or absconding. It applies where a child has been unlawfully taken and kept away from a responsible person named in an emergency protection order or a care order or police protection, or where a child has run away or is missing. The effect of the order is to direct anyone who is able to do so to produce the child or give information regarding the child. A police constable may be authorized to enter premises to search for the child using reasonable force if required.

PRIVATE LAW ORDERS

Private law orders have replaced all the concepts of custody, care and control and can be made by the court without the threshold criteria being satisfied. Section 8 orders cannot be made as a shortcut to obtaining powers otherwise obtainable from care or supervision orders, where these would be better for the child's welfare. However, a Section 8 order may be made as an alternative to a care or supervision order.

General points applying to all Section 8 orders

- Section 8 orders cannot be made in respect of a child over the age of 16 years unless there are 'exceptional circumstances'. These circumstances are not defined, but the Guidance and Regulations give the example of a child who is 'mentally handicapped' (the modern UK English term would be 'learning-disabled'). It is also noted that this confirms established practice under previous legislation, where it is assumed to be pointless to try to compel a child over the age of 16 years to live with someone against their will. (It also, partially at least, brought the law into line with the expectation on 'consent'.)

- Section 8 orders, however, do not lapse automatically at age 16 years.
- The court may add directions as to how any of the Section 8 orders are carried out.
- The court may put conditions on the person or people:
  - in whose favour the order is made;
  - who is the parent with the most parental responsibility;
  - with whom the child is living;
  - to whom the conditions are expressed to apply.
- The court can specify the period for which a Section 8 order applies or for which specific provisions apply.
- The court can add any 'incidental supplemental or consequential provision it sees fit'.
- The paramountcy principle, 'delay-is-prejudicial' principle, 'no-order' presumption and (if opposed) welfare check list all apply.
- Unless limited by legal aid certificates, 'the court' may be a magistrates', county or high court.
- All Section 8 orders are discharged by a care order.
- The court may award costs to discourage unwarranted applications. Also, the court may prohibit further applications.

Residence order

This requires a named child to live with a specific person or people. If they do not already have it, such person(s) then automatically gain 'parental responsibility'. The people named in a residence order do not necessarily have to live at the same address, but, as noted above, specific provisions about the arrangements may be made. There are also additional restrictions on changing a child's surname or removing a child from the UK without written consent or with parental responsibility (the person(s) named on the order may take the child abroad for an unlimited number of periods of less than one month.)

Applications for a residence order may be made *as of right* by:

- any parent, including an unmarried father;
- any person who has a residence order;
- any party to a marriage if the child is a child of the family;
- any person who has lived with the child for more than three years;
- any person who has the consent of all those named on a previous residence order;
- if the child is in care, any person with the consent of the local authority;
- if the child is not in care, any person with parental responsibility.

Anyone else, *including the child*, may be granted a residence order with leave of the court (an exception is a recent foster parent without leave of the local authority, unless he or she is a relative of the child). Appeal against a residence order is to the High Court from the Magistrates' Court, or to the Appeal Court from a county or high court.

A residence order is the only Section 8 order that may be made for a child 'in care', but the local authority itself may not apply.

Section 8 orders may be made for children who are 'looked after' ('accommodated') by the local authority (formerly called 'voluntary care').

Contact order

This is an order that requires a person with whom a child lives to arrange for the child to have contact with another person. Contact is not simply face-to-face contact, but could also include indirect contact (e.g. by telephone or exchange of photographs.)

The application criteria for a contact order are the same as those for a residence order (see above.)

Specific issue order

This is the general order that covers other issues relating to the welfare of the child, over which a person with parental responsibility might decide, e.g. education and medical care. Applicants as of right include those with parental responsibility or with a residence order in respect of the child. Anyone else may apply with leave of the court.

Local authorities may not apply for a specific issue or a prohibited steps order in order to obtain powers that would otherwise be obtained by a care order.

Prohibited steps order

This is the general order that is the counterpart to the specific issues order. It requires a person with parental responsibility to refrain from a specific action without permission of the court. Exact 'prohibited steps' are not specified in the Act but might include particular religious training or medical treatment.

The categories of applicants allowed are the same as those described under 'specific issues' (see above).

Family assistance order (Section 16)

This order replaces the supervision order possible under previous divorce legislation. It is a short-term order (up to six months) intended to smooth periods of transition and the process of divorce. The assistance may be to the child or to the person caring for the child and usually will be of expert input. A social worker or probation officer (acting as a court welfare officer) will be appointed to supervise the carrying out of the order.

CONCLUSION

It is not only those who work directly with children who need to be aware of the law as it relates to younger age groups. There are many situations within the mental health field where it is necessary to consider the implications for child protection, parenting and child welfare. Giving informed opinion in these circumstances would be greatly supported by knowledge of the relevant legislation. Such knowledge, or lack of it, may even affect the credibility of an expert opinion.

REFERENCES

American Academy of Pediatrics (1999). Committee on psychosocial aspects of child and family health: the child in court – a subject review. *Pediatrics* **105**, 1145–8.

American Psychiatric Association (2000). *Diagnostic and Statistical Manual of Mental Disorders*, 4th edn, text revision. Washington, DC: American Psychiatric Association.

Bentovim, A (1991). Significant harm in context. In: Adcock, M, White, R, Hollows, A (eds). *Significant Harm: Its Management and Outcome*. Croydon: Significant Publications, pp. 29–59.

Brophy, J (2001). *Child Psychiatry and Child Protection Litigation*. London: Gaskell.

Clarke Hall, W, Morrison, ACI (1990). *Clarke Hall and Morrison on Children*, 10th edn. *Special Bulletin: A Guide to the Children Act 1989*. London: Butterworths.

Department of Health (1998). *Mental Health Act 1983: Memorandum on Parts 1 to 6, 8 and 10*. London: The Stationery Office.

Department of Health (1999). *Code of Practice to the Mental Health Act 1983*. London: The Stationery Office.

Department of Health (2000). *Framework for the Assessment of Children in Need and Their Families*. London: The Stationery Office. (Also available at www.doh.gov.uk/scg.cin.htm.)

Department of Health (1991). *Working Together Under the Children Act 1989*. London: HMSO.

Mitchels, B, Prince, A (1992). *The Children Act and Medical Practice*. Bristol: Jordan & Sons.

Spencer, JR, Flin, R (1993). *The Evidence of Children*, 2nd edn. London: Blackstone Press.

World Health Organization (1992). *The International Classification of Diseases*, 10th edn. *Classification of Mental and Behavioural Disorders: Clinical Descriptions and Diagnostic Guidelines*. Geneva: World Health Organization.

18

Old age

Most aspects of risk assessment and medicolegal issues related to capacity are covered in previous chapters of this book; this chapter deals with a few remaining aspects of particular relevance to the care of the elderly.

Elderly patients are more likely than younger patients to suffer from dementia. The involuntary detention of such patients with dementia, under the Mental Health Act 1983, poses its own particular difficulties, in so far as it is the case that the legal framework exists to allow, but not require, the compulsory detention of such patients and, conversely, there may exist patients who should be detained against their wishes, in order to protect them against physical harm, but the necessary legislation to implement this course of action does not exist.

DANGEROUSNESS

A key criterion that may allow a patient suffering from dementia to be detained compulsorily under the Mental Health Act 1983 is that of dangerousness. This may be to others or to self.

Dangerousness to others may manifest itself in the following ways, sometimes as a result of atrophy of the frontal lobes, leading to disinhibition:

- physical violence
- indecent exposure
- sexual molestation
- verbal or written threats to others.

Dangerousness to the self may be evidenced as:

- being a fire risk by not switching off heaters, cookers, electric fires, irons, etc. properly;
- being at risk of scalding oneself with hot water, e.g. when trying to bathe without assistance;
- an inability to feed oneself; e.g. in advanced (stage 3) Huntington's disease, it is usually very difficult, if not impossible, for a patient to feed if his or her food has not been liquefied;

■ being at risk of hypothermia as a result of not keeping oneself sufficiently
warm during cold weather;

■ an inability to maintain an adequate degree of hygiene and sanitation,
leading in turn to a risk of life-threatening infection.

In such cases, detention in hospital may need to be only temporary, until
appropriate measures are implemented. For example, a patient with dementia
may be able to return home safely once automatic switches that turn off cookers
and heaters are fitted and regular assistance is provided to help with feeding,
toileting and bathing.

OTHER LEGAL ASPECTS

Dementia also has other legal implications, most of which centre on the question
of capacity. In many cases, the diagnostic classification (mild, moderate or severe
dementia), and reports by psychiatrists and psychologists, may be considered
important by a court. However, if a lawyer finds that a person fulfils the traditional
criteria of having a 'sound disposing mind', then this is usually deemed sufficient
to assume that testamentary capacity has not been affected unduly by dementia.

Dementia may affect the ability of a patient to give consent to treatment and
consent to take part in medical research. These issues are considered further in
Chapter 6 of this book. Matrimonial capacity and contractual capacity may be
affected, as may be the eligibility of the person to adopt a child.

Finally, criminal responsibility may be affected by dementia.

19

People with learning disabilities

INTRODUCTION

Intellectual disability has a rich history of alternative terms in response to changes in public attitudes towards people who suffer with impaired intelligence. The World Health Organization (WHO) has used the concepts of impairment, disability and handicap to denote the loss/abnormality of a physiological/ anatomical/psychological function that leads to loss of an ability normal in human beings and ultimately to the social disadvantage associated with that loss (*Re C* (1994) 1 All ER 819). In current practice, intellectual disability is defined as an event that has occurred during the developmental period and that has led to incomplete or arrested development of the mind that is especially characterized by impairments in adaptive skills and an IQ of less than 70 (American Association on Mental Retardation 1992, American Psychiatric Association 1995, World Health Organization 1992).

In the past in the UK, asylums under the Lunacy Act, poor-law workhouses and idiot asylums accepted all mentally disabled individuals (Thomson 1996, p. 130). However, the **Mental Deficiency Act 1913** made special provisions for people who had a mental deficiency or intellectual disability. The segregational policies persisted until the early 1970s, when they were challenged by the widespread social changes that took place in the second part of the twentieth century. Also, the **Education Act 1971** recognized that all children had a right to education, including those with severe intellectual disability and who, up to that point, were considered to be uneducable. Thus, people with intellectual disability started to leave the asylums and were housed in small supported facilities in the community. The main focus of the new plan was to help people with intellectual disability to participate in 'the mainstream of life, living in ordinary houses in ordinary streets, with the same range of choices as any citizen, and mixing as equals with other, and mostly not handicapped members of their community' (Russell 1997, p. 16).

An important tenet of the changes that occurred following the closure of institutions was that people with intellectual disability have the same rights in law as any other citizen and they should be encouraged to make decisions about their lives. They should be protected from abuse and exploitation, should have a valued role in society, and should enjoy their rights vis-à-vis society's duties towards them. In this chapter, we review the law in its relevance to adults with an intellectual disability in the light of recent changes in legislation in the European Union (EU), including the UK.

CAPACITY TO CONSENT

Consent is the cornerstone of the modern doctor–patient relationship and is, essentially, an ethical doctrine. However, the right to self-determination and the autonomy of competent adults is protected by the law of battery and was expressed thus in *Schloendorff* v. *Society of New York Hospitals* (Kennedy and Grubb 1994, p. 87):

> Every adult person of sound mind has a right to determine what shall be done with his own body; and a surgeon who performs an operation without his patient's consent commits an assault, for which he is liable in damages.

Consent must be informed, i.e. the patient must be given information about his or her condition and the proposed treatment, must have a (broad) understanding of the treatment and of the likely consequences of receiving a different (or even no) intervention, and must make a decision of his or her free will.

The criteria that are used currently to assess capacity to consent to treatment (Eastman criteria) were established in the case of *Re C* (1994), a patient with schizophrenia who refused to have his gangrenous leg amputated. The case emphasized that to be deemed competent, a patient does not always have to accept medical opinion, and a level of self-assessment of the likely consequences of his refusal can be accepted (Raymont 2002). However, in a subsequent case (MB (Caesarean Section) Re (CA) (1997) 2 FLR 426), a pregnant patient was found to be lacking capacity in making a decision about having a caesarean delivery because of a needle phobia and consequent impairment in her mental functioning. The medical intervention was given lawfully in the patient's best interests, as she was likely to suffer more were she not to have had the treatment.

It is a frequent misconception that a person with intellectual disability has limited or no capacity. It is now accepted widely that additional help ought to be provided in encouraging an individual with intellectual disability to communicate his or her wishes by using signs or pictorial materials. A study of ability to consent in people with intellectual disability used three vignettes to examine the impact of verbal fluency and memory on capacity (Arscott et al. 1999). Forty adults were asked whether they understood the presenting problem, the nature of the proposed intervention, the alternative risks and benefits, how they would be involved in deciding, and whether they were able to offer a rationale for treatment. Overall, over three-quarters had some understanding of at least one vignette and one-eighth could process all three vignettes. Abstract issues such as rights, options and consequences of decisions were the most difficult for participants to answer. Strategies that have been considered in improving capacity include attention to communication problems, information presented in accessible form, and treatment of any underlying mental disorder before capacity is assessed (Bellhouse et al. 2001).

No one can consent to treatment on behalf of an adult, even though that adult may have an intellectual disability. For incapacitated adults, the test of 'best interests' is used to judge whether a treatment ethically should be given either in a life-threatening situation or in ordinary care. Bicknell (1989) called carrying out simple tasks of caring by health professionals as 'acting in good faith'.

The test of best interests was introduced in the case of *Re F* v. *West Berkshire Health Authority* (1990) 2 AC 1, (1989) 2 All ER 545 (HL) (sterilization), in which doctors asked for a court decision in order to perform a sterilization operation on an adult woman with severe intellectual disability. It is set in case law that any treatment may be provided to an incompetent adult if it is to save life, is to ensure improvement or prevent deterioration in health, and is in the patient's best interests. The judges applied the 'Bolam standard of best interests' (*Bolam* v. *Friern Hospital Management Committee* (1957) 1 WLR 582), which states that a treatment has been given appropriately if it is in line with current competent medical opinion (see also Brazier 1992 for more information).

Following on from the Mental Incapacity Report (1995), a new definition of incapacity is proposed whereby the person is 'unable by reason of mental disability to make or communicate a decision (where mental disability includes 'any disability or disorder of mind or brain, permanent or temporary, resulting in an impairment or disturbance of mental functioning') (Lord Chancellor's Department 1999, p. 8).

The inability to make a decision is defined as 'inability to understand or retain the information relevant to the decision, or inability to make a decision based on that information (Lord Chancellor's Department 1999, p. 8).

This is similar, but not identical, to the test of incapacity in *Re C* (1994) and *Re MB* (1997), as it leaves out the requirement of belief; therefore, those who make unusual health decisions or experience a transient impaired judgement are not excluded from making their own decisions about their (mental) healthcare. The same principles also guide the framework of the Draft Mental Incapacity Bill (2003). Furthermore, it is recognized that capacity refers to the specific decision that needs to be made and therefore individuals may lack capacity for some matters but not for others. The proposals are far-reaching and aim at enhancing the range of choices and independence of people who are mentally incapacitated through a set of measures that clarify the process of decision-making.

LEGISLATION

Mental Health Act

Mental impairment and severe mental impairment

The **Idiots Act 1886** was the first to provide separate confinement for 'idiots and imbeciles'. Further legislation (1904–08) also provided for many people with inadequate personalities and mild intellectual disability (Hassiotis 1997, p. 56). Mental defect was defined in 1927 as 'a condition of arrested or incomplete development of mind existing before the age of 18 whether arising from inherent causes or induced by disease or injury'. There were four recognized types of mental defect: idiots, imbeciles, feeble-minded and moral defectives. The **Mental Health Act 1959** replaced these grades of cognitive impairment with the terms 'severe subnormality' and 'subnormality'. It recommended uniform procedures for the management of both mental illness and intellectual disability. During the consultations of the review of the 1959 Act, organizations acting on behalf of people with intellectual disability campaigned hard for the term to be taken out of the Act. The root of their argument was that the terminology suggested that people with intellectual disability were always disturbed and, if in need of civil commitment, it was likely to be because of the presence of mental illness. There were fears that once in hospital, adults with intellectual disability would face greater obstacles in obtaining release. The Mental Health Act 1983 set out the following definition of severe mental impairment (Jones 1988, p. 13):

> ... a state of arrested or incomplete development of mind which includes severe impairment of intelligence and social functioning and is associated with abnormally aggressive or seriously irresponsible conduct on the part of the person concerned.

In effect, this definition means that intellectual disability must be associated with such behaviour that places the person or others at risk in order for the patient to be detained. Although this might be considered as an improvement on the previous definition, it has pitfalls in practice, since the degree of impairment may be difficult to ascertain and the system of detaining incompetent individuals in this way has been criticized as relying too much on a medical model despite the safeguards of the Mental Health Act.

Alexander and Singh (1999) found that sections 2 and 3 were the most commonly used in their survey of a tertiary treatment service for adults with intellectual disability. The legal category of mental disorder was used in only half of the admitted patients, although two-thirds had an identifiable mental illness on examination. A review of 55 case notes of adults with intellectual disability who were detained under the Mental Health Act 1983 because of mental illness and severe mental impairment in one district in the UK showed that the majority were young men and resident in an institution (73 per cent) or special hospital (27 per cent) for over 6 years. Twenty-nine per cent were placed under a restriction order and 31 per cent were currently being, or had been, treated for mental disorder (Clarke et al. 1992). All were considered to be a risk to themselves and/or others.

Guardianship orders (Mental Health Act 1983)

Guardianship occasionally has been used to manage adults with intellectual disability in the community who do not engage with services and pose a risk to themselves or others because of personality difficulties or frank mental disorder. Sometimes, these patients may be repeat offenders and guardianship has been perceived as breaching the gap in the lack of probation or appropriate custodial facilities.

Whitworth and Singhal (1995) carried out a retrospective survey of services for people with intellectual disability in four health districts in Merseyside, UK. They found that guardianship orders had been used ten times in 5 years. One of the main problems identified was the inherent difficulty in imposing community supervision under the order. Another concern expressed by clinicians was about the definition of 'seriously irresponsible conduct', because it would exclude patients who had a mild degree of behavioural problems or self-neglect and/or would be overinclusive and thus used in a much wider context. Guardianship orders are generally seen as difficult to implement and offer doubtful benefits to the care of vulnerable adults with intellectual disability and mental disorders.

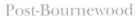

Post-Bournewood

Mr L, a man with severe autism, intellectual disability and epilepsy, had no capacity to consent or communicate his wishes. Following a period of disturbance, he was admitted to a local psychiatric hospital, where he had been an inpatient for many years. His foster carers sought a declaration that he was detained unlawfully, since he could neither consent not dissent to his admission. In the most recent court decision about the case (*Regina* v. *Bournewood Community and Mental Health Trust, Ex Parte L* (1998)), the law lords ruled that Mr L was not detained unlawfully. However, this case throws into focus the complexities of, and gaps in, the current system that leave incapacitated patients who are unable to dissent admitted to hospital informally and whose civil rights maybe compromised (Dickenson and Shah 1999). Eastman and Peay (1998) criticized the use of the doctrine of necessity in such cases, particularly as the boundaries between assent by default and meaningful consent are blurred. For people admitted informally, there is a real worry that their human and civil rights are not protected sufficiently by the Mental Health Act (Dickenson and Shah 1999).

Current issues

The Mental Health Act 1983 is currently being reviewed by the government, and a new draft Bill is now published following the consultation of 2002–03 (see www.doh.gov.uk/policyandguidance/healthandsocialcaretopics/mentalhealth for more information, September 2004). Assessment of capacity is central to the revised Act. It recommends what has been considered good practice for some time, i.e. that assessment for detention should include an evaluation of capacity, that clinical teams should develop advanced agreements with people with chronic mental illness, and that nominated deputies or carers should be consulted in any treatment plans.

Szmukler and Holloway (1998) have called for an Act based on incapacity to avoid further discrimination against psychiatric patients in treatment decisions. However, there are continuing problems that need to be overcome, such as improvement of the process of assessing capacity, increase in research in this area, and ongoing training of medical students and doctors in assessing competence and capacity.

Human Rights Act 1998

The Human Rights Act 1998 came into force on 2 October 2000. It incorporates into UK law the bulk of the substantive rights set out in the European Convention on Human Rights (see also Chapter 22). Individuals can now bring cases for violation of human rights against public bodies in the UK rather than taking their case to the European Court in Strasbourg.

In practice, UK courts and tribunals have to take account of the Human Rights Act and to ensure that the development of the common law is compatible with the Convention rights. However, the way in which the UK courts will interpret the Convention rights, and the impact that these will have on medical decision-making, is not yet known. It is expected that a patient could use the Human Rights Act if he or she found that their expectations of healthcare, including mental healthcare, are not met and in cases of poor standards of care or negligence. Further recommendations for the protection of human rights of detained mentally ill patients have been made by cases brought before the European Court of Human Rights (Department of Health 2004). Detained mentally ill patients have already appealed against their admissions under the provisions of the Human Rights Act 1998 ((2001) EWCA Civ 239; (2001) 98(15) LSG 33; (2001) 145 SJLB. 107).

OFFENDERS WITH INTELLECTUAL DISABILITIES

The issues of criminal responsibility, disposal and diversion in relation to learning disabled offenders have challenged legal systems around the world for centuries. Offenders with intellectual disabilities frequently have limited or no understanding of legal procedure, are vulnerable to making false confessions in police custody (Clare and Gudjonsson 1993, 1995), and cope poorly with prison regimes and other inmates (Murphy and Clare 1998). Low intelligence is one of the factors associated with delinquency, although it is debatable whether rates of criminality among the population with learning disabilities are different from those in the population of average intelligence (Murphy and Mason 1999).

Prevalence rates of suspects with learning disabilities in police stations vary between less than one per cent (Winter et al. 1997) and nearly eight per cent (Gudjonsson et al. 1993), although the decision to test intelligence in the stressful setting of the police station may have led to overestimates in the latter study.

A study of six urban and rural courts in Australia suggests that up to 24 per cent of defendants may have intellectual disabilities (Hayes 1997). However, this study included a high percentage of the Aboriginal population, for whom instruments for psychometric assessment have not been standardized.

Prison studies show rates between no intellectual disabilities at all (Murphy et al. 1995) and 9.5 per cent (Brown and Courtless 1971), but these reports have been criticized on the grounds that their findings may be inaccurate due to the use of different psychometric instruments across studies, poor training of personnel administering the tests, and conditions of testing and diversion procedures in place.

Mason (1998) reported that ten per cent of a sample of offenders on probation orders were identified as having intellectual disabilities.

Types of offending

It has been shown that people with learning disabilities most commonly commit property offences (Day 1993). Sexual offending and fire-setting are, however, the offence categories that traditionally have been most linked with this group, although the nature of the association is unclear (Day 1994, Dorbán et al. 1993, Kearns and O'Connor 1988). Non-sexual aggressive offending is a less common focus of published research.

Sex offenders with learning disabilities have high rates of recidivism, as shown by the group studied by Day (1994), who found that up to 50 per cent had subsequent reconviction for offences other than sex offences. Data from the

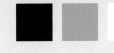
Danish Central Register showed that crimes of property appear to diminish, whilst violence, arson and sexual offences were increasing in offenders with intellectual disability and who had served sentences (Lund 1990).

Legislation for offenders with intellectual disability

The **Police and Criminal Evidence Act (1984)** provided for improved regulation of police interviews of people thought to be mentally disordered by involving the appointment of an 'appropriate adult'. The role of the appropriate adult is to facilitate communication between the police and the arrested person and, if there is no lawyer present, to try to ensure that the interview is conducted fairly. However, an adult has the right to request that an arrested person is legally represented and should always make such a request, especially if the arrested person does not. The scheme has been criticized because of inadequate training of the adult. and he or she may simply act as a passive observer in cases of the 'right to silence' (Evans and Rawstorne 1997). The Criminal Justice and Public Order Act 1994 (England and Wales) altered the wording regarding the 'right to silence' to rectify a perceived imbalance in the criminal justice system in favour of defendants. This has resulted in increased verbal complexity of the police caution. Offenders with intellectual disabilities are now even less likely to understand the caution, which complicates the interview procedure further (Murphy and Clare 1998).

Diversion from custody

The term 'diversion' refers to the process of securing appropriate health and social services for mentally disordered offenders (MDO) at the earliest stage possible. The nineteenth century saw a lengthy debate about the appropriate disposal options for offenders with mental disorder, following the cases of James Hadfield and Daniel McNaughton (Andoh 1993).

The Reed Report (1992) was very clear that mentally disordered offenders should be diverted from prison and that offenders with intellectual disabilities in particular should be placed '... as far as possible in the community, rather than in institutional settings ... and under conditions of no greater security than is justified by the degree of danger they present to others or to themselves'.

Diversion schemes developed over the past decade have focused mainly on the court stage of the Criminal Justice System. Published work in the UK and the USA relating to identification of intellectually disabled offenders in courts indicates that there is poor recognition of intellectual disabilities and, hence, a low chance of offenders to be diverted to suitable services (Hassiotis et al. 2002).

Some individuals who are violent or persistent offenders and with enduring mental health problems will require semi-secure or secure facilities and are likely to be detained under the Mental Health Act 1983 (sections 37 and 41) (Singh et al. 1991).

The **Criminal Procedure (Insanity) Act 1964 (amended 1992)** is intended to protect people who are unfit to plead. The special verdict of not guilty by reason of insanity is used very infrequently nowadays. If an offender with intellectual disability is found unfit to plead, then the end result may still be the special verdict. On both of these occasions, the outcome is indefinite detention under secure conditions. It should be noted that there are other disposal options available (Prins 1990).

There is concern that the civil liberties of offenders with intellectual disability may suffer under new proposals to detain people who as much as express ideas of violence towards people known to them or the public at large. This issue is of particular importance in the USA, where adults with intellectual disability and who have committed serious crimes, i.e. murder, may be subject to the death penalty. Although some have argued against such outcomes given the person's diminished responsibility in the crime, others hold the view that offenders with intellectual disability, taken per case, may indeed be culpable and that to assume otherwise is a violation of their rights to respect and self-determination (Calnen and Blackman 1992).

CONCLUSION

Adults, including offenders, with intellectual disability are subject to the same rules and rights as their peers of normal intelligence. Some advances have already been made in the commitment of mental healthcare agencies to facilitate their integration and full participation in the community. Recent legislation has given people with intellectual disability powers to assert their choices and challenge perceived notions of care by health professionals. The Human Rights Act 1998 will undoubtedly contribute to ensuring that adults with intellectual disability receive proper assessment of their needs.

The Draft Mental Incapacity Bill and the Draft Mental Health Act Bill are genuine efforts to address aspects of the current legal system that have created inequalities in the care of people with intellectual disability. Research into ways in which capacity and consent to treatment can be assessed correctly is paramount so that individuals are less likely to suffer violation of their rights to a free and independent life.

REFERENCES

Alexander, RT, Singh, I (1999). Learning disability and the Mental Health Act. *British Journal of Developmental Disabilities* **45**, 119–22.

American Association on Mental Retardation (1992). *Mental Retardation: Definition, Classification and Systems of Supports.* Washington, DC: American Association on Mental Retardation.

American Psychiatric Association (1995). *Diagnostic and Statistical Manual of Mental Disorders,* 4th edn. Washington, DC; American Psychiatric Association.

Andoh, B (1993). The McNaughton Rules: the story so far. *Medico-Legal Journal* **61**, 93–103.

Arscott, K, Dagnan, D, Kroese, BS (1999). Assessing the ability of people with a learning disability to give informed consent to treatment. *Psychological Medicine* **29**, 1367–75.

Bellhouse, J, Holland, A, Clare, I, Gunn, M (2001). Decision-making capacity in adults: its assessment in clinical practice. *Advances in Psychiatric Treatment* **7**, 294–301.

Bicknell, J (1989). Consent and people with mental handicap. *British Medical Journal* **299**, 1176–7.

Brazier, M (1992). *Medicine, Patients and the Law*. London: Penguin Books.

Brown, BS, Courtless. TF (1971). *The Mentally Retarded Offender*. Publication no. (HSM) 72-90-39. Washington, DC: Department of Health Education and Welfare.

Calnen, T, Blackman, LS (1992). Capital punishment and offenders with mental retardation: response to the Penry Brief. *American Journal on Mental Retardation* **96**, 557–64.

Clare, I, Gudjonsson, GH (1993). Interrogative suggestibility, confabulation, and acquiescence in people with mild learning disabilities (mental handicap): implications for reliability during police interrogations. *British Journal of Clinical Psychology* **32**, 295–301.

Clare, I, Gudjonsson, GH (1995). The vulnerability of suspects with intellectual disabilities during police interviews: a review and experimental study of decision making. *Mental Handicap Research* **8**, 110–28.

Clarke, DJ, Beasley, J, Corbett, JA, Krishnan, VH, Cumella, S (1992). Mental impairment in the West Midlands. *Medicine, Science and the Law* **32**, 225–32.

Day, K (1993). Crime and mental retardation: a review. In: Howells, K, Hollin, C (eds). *Clinical Approaches to the Mentally Disordered Offender*. Chichester: John Wiley & Sons, pp. 111–43.

Day, K (1994). Male mentally handicapped sex offenders. *British Journal of Psychiatry* **165**, 630–9.

Department of Constitutional Affairs (2003). *Draft Mental Incapacity Bill (June 2003)*. London: Department of Constitutional Affairs.

Department of Health (2004). *Equality and Human Rights*. www.dh.gov.uk/policyandguidance/equality&human rights.

Department of Health and Home Office (1983). *The Mental Health Act*. London: The Stationery Office.

Dickenson, D, Shah, A (1999). The Bournewood Judgment: a way forward? *Medical Science and Law* **39**, 280–4.

Dorbán, P, Gunn, J, Holland, T, Kopelman, MD, Robertson, G, Taylor, PJ (1993). Organic disorders, mental handicap and offending. In: Gunn, J, Taylor, P (eds). *Forensic Psychiatry: Clinical Legal and Ethical Issues*. London: Butterworth-Heinemann, pp. 285–328.

Eastman, N, Peay, J (1998). Bournewood: an indefensible gap in mental health law. *British Medical Journal* **317**, 94–5.

Evans, R, Rawstorne, S (1997). Appropriate behaviour. *Community Care* **1181**, 30–1.

Gudjonsson, GH, Clare, I, Rutter, S, Pearse, J (1993). *Persons at Risk During Interview in Police Custody: The Identification of Vulnerabilities.* Royal Commission on Criminal Justice research study no. 12. London: HMO.

Hassiotis, A (1997). Ethical and legal considerations in the care of adults with learning disabilities and psychiatric disorders: clinical practice and research. MA dissertation. London: King's College London.

Hassiotis, A, Barron, P, Banes, J (2002). Offenders with intellectual disabilities: the size of the problems and therapeutic outcomes. *Journal of Intellectual Disability Research* **46**, 454–63.

Hayes, S (1997). Prevalence of intellectual disability in local courts. *Journal of Intellectual and Developmental Disability* **22**, 71–85.

Jones, R (1988). *Mental Health Act Manual,* 2nd edn. London: Sweet and Maxwell.

Kearns, A, O'Connor, A (1988). The mentally handicapped criminal offender. a ten year study of two hospitals. *British Journal of Psychiatry* **152**, 848–51.

Kennedy, I, Grubb, A (1994). *Medical Law: Text With Materials,* 2nd edn. London: Butterworths.

Law Commission Report (1995). *Mental Incapacity.* London: HMSO.

Lord Chancellor's Department (1999). *Making Decisions.* CM4465. London: The Stationery Office.

Lund, J (1990). Mentally retarded offenders in Denmark. *British Journal of Psychiatry* **156**, 726–31.

Mason, J (1998). Identifying and responding to people with learning disabilities in the probation service. PhD thesis. Canterbury: University of Canterbury.

Murphy, G, Harnett, H, Holland, A (1995). A survey of intellectual disabilities amongst men on remand in prison. *Mental Handicap Research* **8**, 81–98.

Murphy, G, Clare, I (1998). People with learning disabilities as offenders or alleged offenders in the UK Criminal Justice System. *Journal of the Royal Society of Medicine* **91**, 178–82.

Murphy, G, Mason, J (1999). People with developmental disabilities who offend. In: Bouras, N (ed.). *Psychiatric and Behavioural Disorders in Developmental Disabilities and Mental Retardation.* Cambridge: Cambridge University Press, pp. 226–45.

Prins, H (1990). Mental abnormality and criminality-an uncertain relationship. *Medical Science and Law* **30**, 247–58.

Raymont, V (2002). 'Not in perfect mind': the complexity of clinical capacity assessment. *Psychiatric Bulletin* **26**, 201–4.

Russell, O (1997). *Seminars in the Psychiatry of Learning Disability.* London: Gaskell.

Singh, TH, Radhakrishnan, G, Richardson, EM (1991). A community-based mental handicap outpatient clinic: a 5-year retrospective study. *Journal of Mental Deficiency Research* **35**, 125–32.

Szmukler, G, Holloway, F (1998). Mental health legislation is now a harmful anachronism. *Psychiatric Bulletin* **22**, 662–5.

Thomson, M (1996). Though ever the subject of psychological medicine: psychiatrists and the colony solution for mental defectives. In: Freeman, H, Berrios, G. (eds). *150 Years of British Psychiatry*, vol. II. London: Athlone, pp. 130–43.

Whitworth, H, Singhal, S (1995). The use of guardianship in mental handicap services. *Psychiatric Bulletin* **19**, 725–7.

Winter, N, Holland, A, Collins, S (1997). Factors predisposing to suspected offending by adults with self reported learning disabilities. *Psychological Medicine* **27**, 595–607.

World Health Organization (1992). *The ICD-10 Classification of Mental and Behavioural Disorders: Clinical Descriptions and Diagnostic Guidelines.* Geneva: World Health Organization.

20

Race, culture and mental health

THE RACE RELATIONS ACT 1976 AND THE RACE RELATIONS ACT 2000

Since April 2001, all public bodies have had a general duty to work towards the elimination of unlawful racial discrimination and to promote equality of opportunity and good relations between different racial groups (Section 1 of the 2000 Act). This duty applies to all those working within the Mental Health Act 1983. There are also important links with the Human Rights Act 1998, which will be considered below.

The Race Relations Act 1976 was designed to strengthen the law against racial discrimination and established a single new statutory body, the Commission for Racial Equality, combining law enforcement and promotional responsibilities in place of the Race Relations Board and Community Relations Commission.

Social service departments were allowed lawfully to discriminate on racial grounds if the need indicated, e.g. appointment of a Vietnamese worker to work with a disabled Vietnamese person. Similarly, discrimination was allowed by employers in training (Section 11 of the Local Government Act 1966 provides funding for special provisions).

Discrimination was made unlawful in employment, education, housing and the provision of goods, facilities and services (including clubs). The provisions were more comprehensive than those of the previous legislation. In particular, the definition of racial discrimination was extended to cover nationality, and it included not only direct discrimination but also the application of unjustifiable requirements and conditions that are formally neutral as between different racial groups but that are, in practice, discriminatory in effect ('indirect' discrimination).

Under the 1976 Act, racial discrimination became a civil wrong for which the normal forms of civil redress are available. Aggrieved individuals are able to seek redress directly in designated county courts or, in employment cases, industrial tribunals.

The Commission for Racial Equality was set up to have general responsibilities for tackling discrimination and promoting equality of opportunity and good race relations.

Section 71 of the Act imposed a general duty on local authorities to take account of the racial dimension in the exercise of their functions. It required local authorities to make appropriate arrangements with a view to ensuring that their various functions are carried out with due regard to the need to eliminate unlawful racial discrimination and to promote equality of opportunity and good relations between people of different racial groups.

Local authorities were encouraged in a related circular (Local Authority Circular 11/77, Race Relations Act 1976, DHSS) to ensure that employment policies and practices should include effective procedures to ensure equality of opportunity for members of minority groups. The Annex to the Circular gave a useful description of the 1976 Act:

> Part I of the Act sets out the definitions of discrimination. In itself it does not define what constitutes unlawful discrimination. This is done in Parts II–IV of the Act, which apply the definitions of discrimination to the contexts of employment, education, housing etc. Exceptions to these provisions are contained in these Parts of the Act. There are also general exceptions (in Part VI), covering such matters as provision to meet special needs, and acts done under statutory authority and other approved arrangements, or to safeguard national security …

> The exception relating to special needs will be of importance to local authorities in the application of their services to minority communities within their area. This exception provides that Parts II–IV of the Act do not render unlawful 'any act done in affording persons of a particular racial group access to facilities or services to meet the special needs of persons of that group in regard to their education, training or welfare, or any ancillary benefits' (Section 35). It is particularly relevant to education, social services and housing. It will for example enable consideration to be given to special housing or social service arrangements where for example particular Asian or West Indian groups have special needs. These may include residential home provision for children and the elderly.

> The Act also permits persons of a particular racial group to be given training for, and to be encouraged to take up, particular work in which no, or relatively few, persons of that racial group have been employed (Section 38).

Discussion

The Race Relations Act was extended to cover nationality, but it does not yet cover religion. This is a problem, and the *Guardian*, on 28 October 1998, noted that the British National Party could attempt to stir up hatred against Muslims without contravening the Public Order Act 1985 on the technicality that Muslims are not a racial group. Note that Sikhs have established themselves in law as a distinct ethnic group, as have Jews, but Rastafarians have not. Gypsies have been given the status of a racial group, but travellers have not. Scots are not a separate ethnic or national group (*Boyce* v. *British Airways* (1997)).

There is a useful analysis in Brayne et al. (2001) on the practical implications of current legislation for workers seeking to practise in an anti-oppressive way.

On 18 February 2001, the *Observer* published figures of race-related crimes, which highlight a major problem in rural areas with small ethnic minority

TABLE 20.1 Racist incidents in parts of England

Constabulary	Size of ethnic minority population	% affected by racist incidents
Northumbria	14 700	7.88
Devon and Cornwall	8900	6.04
Avon and Somerset	25 200	3.52
Dorset	5800	3.19
Gloucestershire	9100	2.84
Hampshire	24 500	2.67
Wiltshire	9200	2.40
London (Met and City)	1 189 300	1.97
West Midlands	287 200	0.54

populations. Table 20.1 is based on figures published in this article. These figures reflect incidents between April 1999 and April 2000.

HUMAN RIGHTS ACT 1998

Article 14 of the European Convention on Human Rights requires that 'the enjoyment of the rights and freedoms set forth in this Convention shall be secured without discrimination on any ground such as sex, race, colour, language, religion, political or other opinion, national or social origin, association with a national minority, property, birth or other status'. It does not provide a free-standing prohibition on discrimination but applies only in relation to the other relevant articles. In a recent European case (*R (on the application of Pretty)* v. *Director of Public Prosecutions* (2001) UKHL 61), Lord Hope held that Article 14 is capable of extending to discrimination in relation to mental capacity. The list of grounds above is illustrative rather than exhaustive; this may prove to be relevant in the light of the European Court case of *HL* v. *UK*, which was published as this book went to press; see preface for comment.

DETAINED PATIENTS FROM BLACK AND MINORITY ETHNIC COMMUNITIES

There is a considerable literature on the overuse of compulsion among certain members of the community. An especially helpful report on the position of detained patients was published by the Sainsbury Centre in 2000. This examined the evidence from a visit by the Mental Health Act Commission to 104 mental health and learning disability units in England and Wales. The visit took place in May 1999 and focused on racial harassment of patients, staff training in race equality and antidiscriminatory practice, and the provision and use of interpreters. The largest group was black Caribbean, comprising 42 per cent of the total. More than two-thirds were men, with the majority aged between 25 and 44 years.

Since 1995, National Health Service (NHS) Trusts have been required to record the ethnicity of all patients admitted; this is also a requirement for any independent hospital providing care for NHS-funded patients. Although all the units surveyed did monitor ethnicity, only exceptionally were the data put to much use.

Three-quarters of the units had no policy for dealing with racial harassment of patients, and two-thirds had no policy on training in race equality and antidiscriminatory practice. However, there were some examples of good practice, which are outlined in the report. Provision of and access to interpreters was variable, and there were still examples of relatives and friends being used as interpreters.

Although the initial report was fairly brief, there were useful contacts for examples of good practice, and the text is recommended strongly as an introduction to this area.

REFERENCES

Brayne, H, Martin, G, Carr, H. (2001). *Law for Social Workers*, 7th edn. London: Blackstone Press.

Sainsbury Centre for Mental Health (2000). *National Visit 2. Improving Care for Detained Patients from Black and Minority Ethnic Communities*. London: The Sainsbury Centre for Mental Health.

21

Mental capacity and international comparison of mental health legislation

INTRODUCTION

At a time when law reform is under consideration, it would seem appropriate to consider mental health law within an international context. It is perhaps surprising that there is so little discussion on this issue in British publications. Other countries can be a source of new ideas as well as being places where lessons may have been learned about ideas that are under consideration, e.g. community treatment orders. Of particular surprise is the lack of attention paid to our closest neighbours in Scotland, Northern Ireland and Ireland. In each of these countries, the law is significantly different from that in England and Wales. This chapter will give a brief description of each of these and will also consider the position in Singapore, the USA and Australia.

This chapter begins with an examination of the law relating to mental incapacity as this frequently overlaps with mental health law. It could indeed be argued that with clear law on mental incapacity, there would be virtually no need for separate mental health legislation. With the possible exception of potential or actual offenders who are seen as a danger to the public, the decision on whether to admit a person to hospital, or to treat a person without his or her consent, could be based on that person's lack of capacity.

LAW REFORM ON MENTAL INCAPACITY

Considerable attention has been paid to this subject in England and Wales for the past ten years but there is no new statute on the books. In 2004, the UK government announced that the Draft Mental Incapacity Bill had received a broadly positive response and that a Mental Incapacity Bill would be introduced by Parliament within the year. Key points of this Bill are listed later in this chapter, following a summary of the historical background to the Bill and of the current legal position on mental incapacity. The Law Commission (1991) published a Consultation Paper on this issue relating to mentally incapacitated adults and decision-making. Paragraph 1.9 of this paper stated:

The existing law relating to decision-making on behalf of mentally incapacitated adults is fragmented, complex and in many respects out of date. There is no coherent concept of their status, and there are many gaps where the law provides no effective mechanism for resolving problems. Debate, stimulated by a series of High Court decisions on sterilisation and abortion, has recently focused on the obtaining of consent to serious medical procedures, but the problems extend far beyond this issue.

Some examples of problem areas identified in the Consultation Paper are:

- consent to medical treatment (this is covered in Chapter 6);
- disputes between relatives;
- significant life decisions: where an adult is not capable of making decisions, such as whether to continue living at home, it is not clear who has ultimate responsibility for making such a decision. Social workers and others sometimes make decisions in a person's best interests, and some cases are referred to the courts for a declaration;
- suspicion of abuse or neglect: it is often not clear when intervention is justified and who should be responsible for taking any action. Since the publication of *No Secrets* (Department of Health 2000), local areas have started to establish vulnerable adult policies. The definition of 'vulnerable adult' is any person over 18 years of age and who is 'unable to take care of him or herself or unable to protect him or herself against significant harm or serious exploitation … [and] … is, or may be, in need of community care services because of mental disorder, physical or learning disability, age or illness' (Law Commission 1995);
- young adults leaving care: despite any mental incapacity, such people may not be eligible for guardianship under the Mental Health Act 1983, and yet neither foster parents nor the local authority will have any continuing legal responsibility under child care law.

THE 1991 REPORT: DECISION-MAKING

The Law Commission listed questions that might arise as to a person's mental capacity to make decisions concerning:

(i) day-to-day living, such as deciding what to eat, what to wear, when to go to bed or get up, whether to have a bath or a haircut; (ii) activities involving more risk, for example, going out alone, crossing roads, participating in sports, going on holiday, making new friends; (iii) major life decisions, such as where to live, whether to enter residential care, whether to get married or have children; (iv) minor routine medical treatment and prophylaxis, such as dentistry, cervical smear tests, vaccinations; (v) major medical treatment which may have advantages and disadvantages, such as the removal of all of someone's teeth and the provision of dentures, or any treatment where the benefits are evenly balanced and a significant degree of choice is involved; (vi) medical treatment necessitating controversial ethical decisions, such as non-therapeutic sterilisation, abortion, tissue donation, cosmetic surgery, participation in medical research or HIV testing; (vii) legal or financial matters, such as claiming benefits, managing money, buying and selling property, making a will.

The law is not always clear as to when some of these decisions can be taken by somebody on behalf of a mentally incapacitated person.

BACKGROUND TO CURRENT LEGISLATION ON INCAPACITY

There is a variety of current legislation that is relevant to these issues, but, as noted above, it is fragmented, complex and, in many respects, out of date. There are some tensions within the law and in its operation. Maximizing freedom and autonomy may conflict with a need for care or control. Again, protection from abuse or exploitation may involve some invasion of a person's autonomy. Another issue is how to identify an acceptable level of risk for an individual. If a professional intervenes without a clear legal base and guidance, then they lay themselves open to allegations of undue influence or misconduct. If a professional does not intervene, then they may be accused of neglecting their duty to care. Finally, not intervening may result in other people being harmed or suffering in some way. If the person causing the harm is seen as 'mentally incapacitated' in some way, then this raises the question of whether he or she should face the full penalty of law (e.g. through a criminal or civil action) or whether he or she should be dealt with differently.

Concept of mental capacity

There is a distinction to be drawn between a legal definition of capacity and incapacity and medical or psychological definitions, although on occasions they will be the same. Paragraph 2.10 of the 1991 paper states:

> A legal incapacity arises whenever the law provides that a particular person is incapable of taking a particular decision, undertaking a particular juristic act, or engaging in a particular activity.

Incapacity can arise from a variety of conditions; historically, these included being under the age of majority, being a married woman, or being of unsound mind. Under modern law, a great many different approaches have developed to the question of capacity based on mental state. Generally, there is a presumption that the person is capable until proved otherwise, and capacity is judged in relation to the particular decision, transaction or activity involved. There is also a basic common-law test of capacity, to the effect that the person concerned must at the relevant time understand in broad terms what he or she is doing and the likely effects of his or her action. Thus, in principle, legal capacity depends upon understanding rather than wisdom, i.e. the quality of the decision is irrelevant as long as the person understands what he or she is deciding. However, this test varies according to specific circumstances. For example, the Mental Health Act contains three approaches:

- one governs compulsory admission to hospital and guardianship (parts II and III);
- one governs consent to treatment for mental disorder (Part IV); and
- one governs decisions relating to property and affairs (Part VII).

Current legal position

There are differences in law according to the area in question.

Compulsory admission to hospital and guardianship

The tests here are not of mental capacity but of the person's mental state and the need for assessment or treatment.

Decisions regarding property and affairs

Under Section 94(2) of the Mental Health Act 1983, powers of the Court of Protection are exercisable when the court is satisfied, after considering medical evidence, that 'a person is incapable, by reason of mental disorder, of managing and administering his property and affairs' (see Chapter 13).

Contracts

The relevant test is whether a person is capable of understanding the general nature of what he or she is doing. The degree of understanding required depends on the nature of the transaction; the more important the transaction, the higher the level of understanding needed. Unless the person is subject to the Court of Protection's jurisdiction, a contract is binding on that person if the other party reasonably believed that the individual was mentally capable at the time of the transaction. This applies even if the person was not so capable.

Wills

To be seen as capable of making a will, a person needs not only to pass the basic test of understanding the nature of the act and its broad effects but also to be able to recall the extent of his or her property and to have an awareness of the moral obligations owed to relatives and others. A person who is mentally disordered may make a legitimate will (even if subject to jurisdiction of the Court of Protection) if it is made during a lucid interval or where delusions have not influenced the disposal of property.

Medical treatment

The basic common-law principle is that everyone's body is inviolate. Any intentional touching may amount to a trespass or battery if it takes place without consent. Thus, any medical procedure involving touch and performed without consent is a tort. There are a number of exceptions, the principal one of which, in relation to medical treatment, is the doctrine of necessity. Necessity provides a justification for medical treatment that would otherwise be a battery. A doctor is entitled to carry out such emergency treatment as is necessary to preserve the life and health of an unconscious patient, notwithstanding that the person is unable to give or withhold consent; indeed, the doctor probably has a duty to do so. Consent to medical treatment, as a defence to an action for battery, can be effective if the patient's consent is 'real', in the sense that he or she understands in broad terms what is involved. Doctors may be liable in negligence if they do not fulfil the duty of care owed to their patients. This duty would include, in addition to the obligation to exercise professional care and skill in diagnosis and treatment, an obligation to advise patients, inform them about treatment, and warn them of any significant risks of treatment (see Chapter 6).

Mental Capacity Bill

A Draft Mental Incapacity Bill was published in June 2003 and was subject to pre-Legislative Scrutiny by a Joint Parliamentary Committee. The government then announced its intention to introduce a revised Mental Capacity Bill within the year.

The Mental Capacity Bill will provide a statutory framework for the protection of vulnerable people, carers and professionals. In response to the lack of clarity identified earlier in this chapter, it should identify who can take decisions in which situations and how they should go about this.

In line with the recommendations from the Law Commission, the Bill states that a person is presumed to have capacity until shown otherwise. It also requires that all practical steps should be taken to help a person make a decision by being given the help and support he or she needs to make and express a choice. People will retain the right to make what might be seen as eccentric or unwise decisions.

Under the provisions of the Bill, if a person were deemed to lack capacity for a particular decision, then there would not be a presumption that he or she lacked capacity for other decisions.

Where a person lacks capacity, all decisions must be made in the person's best interests, with due regard being given to the decision being what the person themselves would have wanted. Decisions made on the behalf of someone else should be the least restrictive of their basic rights and freedoms.

Department of Health fact sheet

In April 2004, the Department of Health published a fact sheet on the proposed Bill. As background information to the Bill, it stated:

> At some point in their lives, millions of people in the UK lose their ability to make decisions that affect their lives – either through illness, disability or injury. And some people are born with disabilities that affect their capacity to make decisions.

> Up to 2 million people are affected by a lack of capacity. For example:

> - Over 700,000 people in the UK currently suffer from dementia and this figure is likely to increase to about 840,000 by 2021.
> - Around 145,000 adults in England have severe and profound learning disabilities and at least 1.2 million have mild to moderate disability. In

Wales over 12,000 people were registered as having a learning disability in 2001.

- 10–15 people per 100,000 of the population will suffer a severe head injury each year, and there are currently an estimated 120,000 people in the UK suffering from the long-term effects of severe brain injury.
- At some point in their lives approximately 1 per cent of the UK population will suffer from schizophrenia, 1 per cent will be subject to manic depression and 5 per cent will have serious or clinical depression.

What the Bill does

The Bill enshrines in law the current best practice. It will provide a legal basis in the following ways:

Best interests

Incapacitated people will be placed at the heart of the decision-making process, and their best interests are key to the whole Bill. The Bill will provide a checklist of factors that decision-makers must work through in deciding what is in a person's best interests.

General authority

This provides the legal basis for a person to act on behalf of an adult who lacks capacity. The Bill will clarify that a person acting under the 'general authority' does not have a new authority to intervene in the life of someone who lacks capacity, but that this protects carers from liability when they act in the best interests of a person who cannot consent. The 'general authority' will be renamed, as there have been concerns about how this might be interpreted.

Lasting powers of attorney

Lasting powers of attorney (LPA) will be established, allowing people to appoint an attorney to act on their behalf if they should lose capacity in the future. A person can choose to apply the LPA to welfare, healthcare and financial matters.

Court-appointed deputies

The Bill will create a system of court-appointed deputies to replace and extend the current system of receivership in the Court of Protection. Deputies will be able to take decisions on welfare, healthcare and financial matters, as determined by the court.

Advance decisions

This will confirm the legal basis for people to make a decision to refuse treatment if they should lose capacity in the future. The Bill sets out the circumstances in which advance decisions may be followed by doctors, together with safeguards that will seek to ensure that the person making the decision was informed fully and that the decision has not changed over time.

Criminal offence

The Bill introduces a new criminal offence of neglect or ill treatment that can be used against anyone who has ill-treated or wilfully neglected a person who lacks capacity. A person found guilty of such an offence may be liable to a term of up to two year's imprisonment.

New Court of Protection

The Bill will establish a new court with jurisdiction to consider applications for financial decisions and serious healthcare cases (such as decisions to undertake irreversible treatments, e.g. sterilization), which are currently dealt with by the High Court. The practical working of the court will be designed around the needs of the person lacking capacity.

New Public Guardian

The Public Guardian will be the registering authority for LPAs and deputies. He or she will supervise deputies appointed by the court and provide information to help the court make decisions. The Public Guardian will register LPAs and, working with other agencies such as the police and social services, will respond to any concerns raised about the way in which the LPA is being operated by the donee(s).

Code of Practice

This will provide guidance on working and dealing with people who lack capacity. A draft outline of the Code will be available to Parliament at the Committee stage of the Bill.

What the Bill does not do

The Bill does not change the law regarding the following:

- Euthanasia: this is, in any case, not a legal concept. It will remain unlawful to take a person's life, in all the same circumstances as now. The Bill will make this explicit.
- Withdrawal of artificial nutrition and hydration (ANH) when a person is in a permanent vegetative state (PVS).

Most of this material is based on the Law Commission's proposals and generally has been received well by those working with people who lack capacity to make certain decisions. The plethora of recent case law in this area can be seen as an indication that statutory reform is needed urgently. England and Wales are already lagging behind Scotland, whose legal changes in this area are considered in the next part of this chapter.

SCOTLAND

Adults With Incapacity (Scotland) Act 2000

Scotland is especially interesting, because the process of law reform has been taking place at the same time as in England and Wales. The first major difference was that Scotland went ahead with an Act to provide for decisions to be made on behalf of adults who lack capacity to make decisions for themselves. This might be due to mental disorder or due to an inability to communicate. Decisions could be about the person's property or financial affairs or (and this is where the law departs from that in England and Wales) about their personal welfare, including medical treatment.

The definition of mental disorder is mental illness or mental handicap. As a result of a reform in 1999, mental illness includes personality disorder. In terms of exclusions, people should not be regarded as mentally disordered by reason solely of immoral conduct, sexual deviancy or dependency on alcohol or drugs, although people whose mental faculties are impaired due to past alcohol or drug abuse do fall within the definition. The Act does not cover people who simply act imprudently.

Sheriffs (the nearest equivalent being magistrates in England and Wales) are given wide powers under the Act. They can make one-off orders (e.g. as to whether property should be sold) and may give directions to anyone acting as an attorney or guardian for someone.

A new post of Public Guardian was created by the Act. The role of the Public Guardian is to supervise people exercising financial powers under the Act and to investigate complaints. The Public Guardian liaises with the Mental Welfare Commission and the relevant local authority, where there might be a common interest.

The Mental Welfare Commission's role was expanded by the Act to include visiting people incapacitated by mental disorder (as opposed to sensory loss) and to investigate complaints. Local authorities have a major role in looking after people with incapacity and to monitor the actions of welfare guardians.

Perhaps the single biggest change was to allow welfare powers of attorney. While mentally capable, an individual can grant, in writing, continuing powers of attorney for welfare matters, including medical treatment.

Mental Health (Scotland) Bill 2002

At the time of writing, this had not been enacted, but it is important for two main reasons: (i) there is a clearer commitment to making it law and (ii) the Bill is significantly different from the equivalent Draft Bill for England Wales. It is, nonetheless, contentious in its own right. Although the covering letter to the Bill states that there are still exclusions (relating to substance misuse, sexual orientation or behaviour, and antisocial or imprudent behaviour), these are not actually listed in the Bill. Personality disorders are included.

The Mental Welfare Commission retains its right to discharge patients despite the introduction of tribunals. It has a duty to visit patients, a power to make inquiries and a general duty to monitor the operation of the Act and to promote best practice.

The Mental Health Tribunal takes over the role of the Sheriff, who currently makes decisions about long-term detention and guardianship.

It is intended to allow patients to make advanced statements, which must be taken into account if any restrictive measures are being sought. This is an example of the impact of having an Act covering incapacity. Another example is the disappearance of guardianship from mental health law and its replacement in the incapacity legislation.

THE MENTAL HEALTH (NORTHERN IRELAND) ORDER 1986

A particular area of interest here is the definition of mental disorder, which excludes personality disorder. Mental illness is defined in Article 3 as 'a state of mind which affects a person's thinking, perceiving, emotion or judgement to the extent that he requires care or medical treatment in his own interests or the interests of other persons'. If a person is detained for a period of up to 28 days, but not beyond, then the assessment period may be disregarded for certain purposes (e.g. disclosures on health for job purposes). Applications for assessment periods always precede longer-term detention (as is being proposed in England and Wales) and can be by an approved social worker (ASW) or nearest relative. The proportion of applications made by ASWs has increased significantly in recent years. (For more on the role of ASWs in Northern Ireland, see Britton et al. 1999.)

THE IRISH MENTAL HEALTH ACT 2001

A particular feature of the very recent Irish law reforms is that a potential patient suffering only from a personality disorder cannot be detained compulsorily. Mental disorder is defined as mental illness, severe dementia or significant intellectual disability.

Applications for involuntary admission can be made by a patient's spouse, a relative, an authorized officer, a Garda or any other person. An admission order is for up to 21 days and can be followed by a further order of up to three months, then six months, and then annually. Tribunals are appointed by the Mental Health Commission and review the use of compulsion. A patient may appeal a tribunal decision to the Circuit Court.

SINGAPORE: MENTAL DISORDERS AND TREATMENT ACT

Singapore is interesting in that it is an example of a country where doctors are given considerable powers to act without reference to another body. A mentally disordered person is someone of unsound mind who is incapable of managing him- or herself or his or her affairs. An initial order for detention of a person of unsound mind for up to 72 hours can be made by a doctor in a psychiatric hospital. If another medical officer at the hospital sees the patient and signs an order, then the patient can be detained for up to one month. Within one month, the person must be seen by two medical officers, who can sign an order of up to one year if it is necessary in the interests of that person's health or safety or for the protection of others. Hospital visitors have specific powers and refer longer-term detained patients to magistrates, who can make further orders. Visitors also have a role in granting leave of absence.

THE USA

Mental health legislation varies from state to state in the USA. However, there are certain common themes. In an important case in 1975 (*O'Connor* v. *Donaldson* (1975) Supreme Court), the Supreme Court ruled that states cannot constitutionally confine a person who is not dangerous and who can live on his or her own or with the help of others. Most states adopted the principle of seeking 'the least restrictive environment' (a phrase that some think, incorrectly, is included in the English and Welsh Mental Health Act). An example is Missouri, where the law was amended in 1978 to try to balance a person's rights with the ability to get services. There needed to be a physical threat or harm caused by the mental illness before a person could be detained. This approach is currently under review, with concerns over the numbers of untreated mentally ill people in the community. Other states have adopted a more rigorous approach to the idea of community treatment, with financial benefits being linked with acceptance of medication and other treatment.

COMMUNITY TREATMENT ORDERS: AN AUSTRALIAN EXAMPLE

Law is state-based in Australia. Under the South Australia Mental Health Act 1993, it is possible to make treatment orders that allow for compulsory treatment in the community. The Guardianship Board can make orders for set periods of up to one year. A community treatment order requires that a person has a mental illness that is amenable to treatment; that a medical practitioner has authorized treatment, which the person has refused or failed to undergo (or is likely to refuse or fail to accept); and that the person should be given the treatment for the illness in the interests of his or her own health and safety or for the protection of others. Treatment cannot include electroconvulsive therapy (ECT). If a person does not comply with a treatment order, then he or she can be conveyed to a treatment centre.

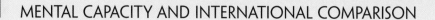

REFERENCES

Britton, F, Campbell, J, Hamilton, B, Hughes, P, Manktelow, R, Wilson, G (1999). *A Study of Approved Social Work in Northern Ireland.* Belfast: DHSS Northern Ireland.

Department of Health (2000). *No Secrets.* London: The Stationery Office.

Law Commission (1991). *Mentally Incapacitated Adults and Decision-Making: An Overview.* London: HMSO.

Law Commission (1995). *Mental Incapacity.* London: HMSO.

FURTHER READING

Department of Constitutional Affairs (2004). *Fact Sheet on Mental Incapacity Bill.* London: Department of Constitutional Affairs. (Also available at www.dca.gov.uk.)

Department of Constitutional Affairs (2004). *The Government's Response to the Scrutiny Committee's Report on the Draft Mental Incapacity Bill.* London: Department of Constitutional Affairs. (Also available at www.dca.gov.uk.)

Department of Health (1997). *Who Decides?* London: The Stationery Office.

22

The Human Rights Act 1998

This Act became operational on 2 October 2000. The delay was to allow judges and others to be trained in how to operate the new legislation. The European Convention on Human Rights (ECHR) was part of a post-Second World War attempt to establish certain basic human freedoms in law. The Act was a major constitutional reform, but it does not remove the sovereignty of Parliament. A court may not strike down primary legislation that is inconsistent with the Convention. However, a court may make a Declaration of Incompatibility, which may lead to a speedy change in the statute. An example of this in relation to Section 72 of the Mental Health Act is considered below. The Act does not incorporate the whole of the European Convention on Human Rights into English law, but it does include the following (the comments refer to some of the recent case law relevant to the mental health field):

ARTICLE 2 RIGHT TO LIFE

Everyone's right to life shall be protected by law. No one shall be deprived of his life intentionally save in the execution of a sentence of a court following his conviction of a crime for which this penalty is provided by law.

This means more than the state refraining from intentional and unlawful taking of life. It also means that public authorities must take appropriate steps to safeguard the lives of people within their jurisdictions (*Edwards* v *United Kingdom* (2002) 35 EHRR 19). People in custody are in a vulnerable position, and authorities have a duty to protect them.

ARTICLE 3 PROHIBITION OF TORTURE

No one shall be subjected to torture or to inhuman or degrading treatment or punishment.

In *A v. United Kingdom* (1999) 27 EHRR 611, the European Court of Human Rights held that states need 'to take measures designed to ensure that individuals within their jurisdiction are not subjected to torture or inhuman or degrading treatment or punishment, including such ill-treatment administered by private individuals'. Key issues are whether the authorities were aware, or ought to have been aware, of abuse and whether they then took reasonable steps to protect people from that abuse. Authorities are under an obligation to protect the health of people deprived of their liberty, and lack of appropriate medical treatment may breach Article 3 (*Keenan* v. *United Kingdom* (2003) 36 EHRR 31). Courts have so far been reluctant to categorize any psychiatric treatment as inhuman and degrading.

ARTICLE 4 PROHIBITION OF SLAVERY AND FORCED LABOUR

ARTICLE 5 RIGHT TO LIBERTY AND SECURITY OF PERSON

No one shall be deprived of their liberty except for specific cases and in accordance with procedure prescribed by law e.g. after conviction, lawful arrest on suspicion of having committed an offence, lawful detention of person of unsound mind, to prevent spread of infectious diseases. Everyone deprived of liberty by arrest or detention shall be entitled to take proceedings by which the lawfulness of the detention shall be decided speedily by a court and release ordered if the detention is not lawful.

In *R (on the application of H)* v. *Mental Health Review Tribunal, North and East London Region (2001) EWCA Civ 415*, the Court of Appeal made a declaration of incompatibility in relation to sections 72 and 73 of the Mental Health Act. This was then addressed by the Mental Health Act 1983 (Remedial) Order 2001 (SI2001/3712), which reversed the burden of proof at tribunals. The grounds for continued detention at a tribunal in effect now mirror the grounds at the first point of detention. The onus is no longer on the patient to demonstrate that he or she does not meet the grounds, and this puts the burden of evidence on the detaining authority.

Several cases have focused on the delays that occur in holding Mental Health Review Tribunal hearings. They should be heard within eight weeks of application, or earlier, depending on the specific features of the case. This has put considerable pressure on the organization of hearings, and at the time of writing there were still significant problems in this area.

ARTICLE 6 RIGHT TO A FAIR TRIAL

Everyone is entitled to a fair and public hearing within a reasonable time by an independent and impartial tribunal.

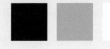

The principles of this article are often extended to psychiatric patients covered by Article 5.4. Keeping information from a patient in a Mental Health Review Tribunal report may be seen to breach the right to a fair trial, even if done to respect Article 8. Staff need to be careful about suggesting this and, if doing so, should certainly relate this to the tribunal rules. A fair hearing has been seen by the European Court as giving a person a right to adversarial proceedings, having a hearing within a reasonable time, equality of arms, knowing the grounds on which a decision is based and access to information necessary to bring the case effectively. Fairness is the essence.

ARTICLE 7 NO PUNISHMENT WITHOUT LAW

ARTICLE 8 RIGHT TO RESPECT FOR PRIVATE AND FAMILY LIFE

Everyone has the right to respect for his private and family life, his home and his correspondence.

There is a dilemma if an approved social worker is obliged by statute to consult with a nearest relative and where this may cause distress to a patient. Consulting when the patient has asked for this not to happen may be seen to breach Article 8. See the discussion in Jones (2002) on the 'practicability' of contacting a nearest relative. Jones suggests that this should be interpreted broadly in the light of the European Convention on Human Rights so that contact could be seen to be impracticable. Staff may wish to seek legal advice. There may be other issues of confidentiality plus the question of children's visits to hospital. The government has failed to act on the *JT* v. *United Kingdom (2000)* case in which they reassured the European Commission that the breach of patients' rights in relation to nearest relatives would be addressed. As a result, Maurice Kay J has made a declaration of incompatibility in relation to Section 26 of the Mental Health Act (*R (on the application of M)* v. *Secretary of State for Health* (2003) All ER 672). Apart from the removal of the nearest relative in the redrafted Mental Health Bill, there has still been no action on this issue, which causes distress to the many people affected by it.

ARTICLE 9 FREEDOM OF THOUGHT, CONSCIENCE AND RELIGION

An inpatient may have restricted access to be able to 'manifest his religion or belief, in worship, teaching, practice and observance'.

ARTICLE 10 FREEDOM OF EXPRESSION

A patient may consider that his or her right to free speech is being denied.

ARTICLE 11 FREEDOM OF ASSEMBLY AND ASSOCIATION

ARTICLE 12 RIGHT TO MARRY

Men and women of marriageable age have the right to marry and to found a family.

A patient may seek conjugal provisions in a secure ward.

ARTICLE 14 PROHIBITION OF DISCRIMINATION

Enjoyment of the rights and freedoms set forth in this Convention shall be secured without discrimination on any ground such as sex, race, colour, language, religion, political or other opinion, national or social origin, association with a national minority, property, birth or other status.

ARTICLE 16 RESTRICTIONS ON POLITICAL ACTIVITIES OF ALIENS

ARTICLE 17 PROHIBITION OF ABUSE OF RIGHTS

ARTICLE 18 LIMITATION ON USE OF RESTRICTION ON RIGHTS

Some articles of the Convention's protocols are also incorporated, such as peaceful enjoyment of possessions, right to education and right to free elections.

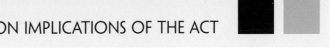

ADVICE ON IMPLICATIONS OF THE ACT

Section 3 of the Act states: 'so far as it is possible to do so, primary legislation and subordinate legislation must be read and given effect in a way which is compatible with the Convention rights'. It does not, however, affect the validity, continuing operation or enforcement of any incompatible primary legislation.

Mental Health Act

The revised Code of Practice to the Mental Health Act 1983 came into effect on 1 April 1999. Although it was drafted before the passing of the Human Rights Act, the Code does make reference to the European Convention in the following passage, which is from Paragraph 1.1 of the Code: 'people to whom the [Mental Health] Act applies (including those being assessed for possible admission) should receive recognition of their basic human rights under the European Convention on Human Rights'. Staff may wish to ask for guidance on the implications of this both in specific instances and as a matter of general principle. Managers and legal sections can expect to become increasingly involved in this area.

A useful source of information on the Human Rights Act 1998 and the European Convention is Wadham and Mountfield (1999). For a broader approach and links with other law, see Wallington and Lee (1999).

Public authorities

Public authorities are required to act in a way that is compatible with ECHR rights unless they are prevented from doing so by statute. Advice from the Department of Health would suggest that the following would be seen as public authorities:

- courts;
- tribunals;
- National Health Service (NHS) Trusts;
- private- and voluntary-sector contractors undertaking public functions under NHS contract;
- local authorities (including social services);
- Primary Care Trusts;
- general practitioners (GPs), dentists, opticians and pharmacists when undertaking NHS work;
- bodies with public functions, such as the General Medical Council (GMC).

The Sainsbury Centre (2000) states that the following probably would be seen to be public authorities:

- Mental Health Act Commission
- National Institute for Clinical Excellence (NICE)
- Commission for Health Improvement
- Health Service Ombudsman.

KEY TERMS

Absolute rights: cannot be limited or qualified (e.g. Article 3 does not ever allow torture or inhuman or degrading treatment).

Limited rights: specify limitations (e.g. the right to liberty allows for the detention of 'persons of unsound mind').

Qualified rights: sets out when interference with such rights is permissible (where in accordance with the law, necessary in a democratic society, related to tone of the aims in the relevant article).

Proportionality: interference with rights must be no more than necessary to achieve the intended objective.

Living instrument: the European Court will interpret the ECHR in light of present-day conditions.

Margin of appreciation: describes the measure of discretion given to the state in deciding on action under scrutiny (e.g. national security).

Positive obligations: many articles expect positive action as well as non-interference with rights.

Declarations of incompatibility: may be made by higher courts, with the expectation that legislation will then be amended to make it compatible with the ECHR.

REFERENCES

Jones R, (2002). *Mental Health Act Manual*, 8th edn. London: Sweet and Maxwell.

Sainsbury Centre (2000). *Briefing 12: An Executive Briefing on the Implications of the Human Rights Act 1998 for Mental Health Services.* London: The Sainsbury Centre for Mental Health.

Wadham, J, Mountfield, H (2001). *Human Rights Act 1998*, 2nd edn. London: Blackstone Press.

Wallington, P, Lee, R (1999). *Statutes on Public Law and Human Rights*, 9th edn. London: Blackstone Press.

SOME KEY RECENT MENTAL HEALTH CASES (2000 TO AUGUST 2004)
(summarized by Paul Barber, Consultant with Bevan Ashford, Solicitors)

1. **Compulsory Treatment/Withdrawal of Treatment Cases**
    (a) *Re SL* (Adult Patient: Sterilization) (Consent, Treatment) (2000) 3 WLR 1288

    This case concerned the request for court authority for a laparoscopic subtotal hysterectomy of a 28-year-old woman suffering severe learning difficulties. The request was based on the woman's heavy menstrual bleeding, which she did not understand, and on the argument that it would have been highly detrimental for her to become pregnant. Rather surprisingly the Judge at first instance authorized the procedure even though sterilization was not the first choice of treatment of the doctors caring for her. However, the Court of Appeal reversed this decision, finding that first, the expert evidence was in favour of a less invasive procedure (insertion of a Mirena coil), even though this would require repeated intervention. A disabled person had the right not to have drastic surgery imposed upon her unless and until it had been demonstrated to be in her best interests. Second, best interests here dictated that the less invasive procedure should have been adopted first and, if it failed, it would have been appropriate to return to seek a declaration in respect of the proposed surgery. The Court clearly felt that the proposed procedure was disproportionate to the medical problem posed. Law Justice Thorpe stated that the judge must have regard to the patient's welfare as the paramount consideration. It is important that when considering what constitutes the patient's best interests (which justifies clinical intervention) the clinician must look beyond mere clinical issues. Although not yet enacted, the 'best interests checklist' proposed in the government's document 'Making Decisions' should be referred to by clinicians so that the process of decision-making has some structure rather than simply relying upon the somewhat circular support of a Bolam-competent body of colleagues.

    (b) *Re A* (Male Sterilization) (2000) 1 FLR 549

    In this case a mother's application for the sterilization of her son who suffered from Down's Syndrome was refused by the Court of Appeal, which held that in the case of a man who is mentally incapacitated, neither the birth of a child nor disapproval of his conduct was likely to impinge on him to a significant degree other than in exceptional circumstances. There was a risk that without sterilization his freedom might be restricted and consequently his quality of life diminished and in individual cases this risk or other risks might weigh in the balance and lead the Court to approve such an operation in other circumstances. The case again emphasizes that it is what is in the patient's best interests (rather than those of the carer) that should determine the outcome.

    (c) *NHS Trust A* v. *M* and *NHS Trust B* v. *H* (2000) 1 All ER 801

    These two cases were the first to consider whether the House of Lords ruling in the Bland case could survive the advent of the Human Rights Act 1998. In all respects the existing law was upheld and declarations given that it would be lawful for artificial feeding to be withdrawn from the two permanent vegetative state (PVS) patients. The Court held that an omission to provide treatment by the medical team would only be incompatible with Article 2 (The Right to Life) where the circumstances are such as to impose a positive obligation on the State to take steps to prolong a patient's life; however, Article 2 only imposed a positive obligation to give life-sustaining treatment in circumstances where, according to responsible medical opinion, such treatment is in the best interests of the patient. It does not impose an absolute obligation to treat if such treatment would be futile; it is doubtful whether families of PVS patients have rights under Article 8 (Respect for Private and Family Life…) separate from the rights of the patient; finally the withdrawal of treatment from PVS patients, being in accordance with the practice of a responsible body of medical opinion, and for a benign purpose in accordance with the best interests of the patients, is legitimate and does not amount to 'degrading treatment' under Article 3; moreover, Article 3 requires the victim to be aware of the inhuman and degrading treatment which he/she is experiencing, or at least to be in a state of physical or mental suffering.

(d) *R v. Collins & Ashwood Hospital Authority Ex Parte Brady* (2000) Lloyd's Rep Med 355

This is the case concerning Ian Brady, who was challenging a decision of his Responsible Medical Officer to force feed him under Section 63 of the Mental Health Act and affirmed the previous law on the subject. Where a patient was suffering from a mental disorder and a hunger strike was deemed to be a manifestation of that illness, Section 63 applied to the circumstances surrounding the commencement and continuation of force feeding as medical treatment for the mental disorder. Brady was incapacitated in relation to his decisions which empowered the RMO to supply medical treatment to him in his best interests. Of course had Brady had capacity and had the force feeding, as medical treatment, not been for the mental disorder from which he was suffering, then he would have been in the same position as, for example, prisoners who have capacity and, like ordinary members of the public, cannot be force fed. Interestingly, the Human Rights Act cases in Strasbourg would in fact permit the force feeding of competent prisoners against their will on the basis of Article 2, but would not require it. In those circumstances there would be an apparent conflict between Article 2 (The Right to Life), and Article 3 (The Right Not To Receive Inhuman Or Degrading Treatment).

(e) *Ms B v. An NHS Hospital Trust* (2002) 2 All ER 449

This widely reported case involved a 43-year-old woman who applied to the Court for a declaration that she had the mental capacity to elect to refuse continuing medical treatment in the form of artificial ventilation. The case was not about what was in her best interests, which only arises where capacity is lacking. The Court, in granting the declaration, made a number of points, but no new law.

(i)   There is a presumption of capacity.

(ii)   An adult of sound mind is entitled to refuse medical treatment even if the doctors believe her to be acting irrationally.

(iii)   While the issue of capacity is being decided the doctors should treat according to best interests principles.

(iv) In the present case the issue was whether Ms B's apparent capacity was overridden by ambivalence, a depressive illness or a failure to try rehabilitation options, and the unnatural surroundings of an ICU.

(v) Once the *Re C* test of capacity was met the doctors were duty bound to follow her wishes not just in refusing new therapies but in discontinuing existing treatment.

(vi) The doctors treating her could not be compelled to switch off the ventilator but would then have a duty to refer her to someone who would.

(vii) In cases of doubt about capacity, where an approach was to be made for outside expertise this should if possible be a joint approach, with the patient fully involved in the process.

(viii) If doubt continued the Official Solicitor could be approached for advice, or an application made to the court which would not decide if the patient should live or die, but whether she had legal capacity. In any event the hospital should not delay resolving the issue.

Note. This case differs from that of Dianne Pretty, where the issue was whether it would be lawful to take active steps to assist in her suicide rather than respect for an adult of sound mind's decision to refuse continuing medical treatment. Ms B has now died, having been taken off the ventilator at her request.

(f) *R (Ex Parte Wooder)* v. *Feggetter* (2002) EWCA Civ 554; (2002) 3 WLR 591
A Second-Opinion Appointed Doctor (SOAD) who certifies under Section 58 of the Mental Health Act that a detained patient should be given medication against his will should give his reasons in writing and these should be disclosed to the patient unless the SOAD or RMO considered that this would be likely to cause serious harm to the physical or mental health of the patient or any other person.

(g) *R v. Ashworth Hospital Authority, ex parte B* (2003) 4 All ER 319
Section 63 of the Mental Health Act provides one of the few occasions when a competent person's refusal to accept medical treatment can be overridden. It provides that the consent of a patient shall not be required for any medical treatment given to him for the mental disorder from which he is suffering...if the treatment is given by or under the direction of the RMO. This case shows the limits to the use of this power. In particular Section 63 does not apply to treatment for *any* mental disorder from which the patient is suffering while liable to be detained but only to the disorder for which he has been classified. So here it was not lawful to treat a patient under Section 63 for psychopathic disorder as the classified disorder was mental illness. If the patient suffered from more than one disorder he would need to be classified accordingly. If treatment was intended for a disorder for which he was not classified the patient would need first to be reclassified, under sections 16, 20 or 72 of the Mental Health Act.

(h) *R v. GMC, ex parte Burke*
Although this case is only at first instance, and may well go to the Court of Appeal, it takes the issues raised in *NHS Trust A* v. *M* at 1(c) above in a rather different direction. It arose from the Applicant's judicial review of the GMC guidance on withholding and withdrawing life prolonging treatments. In

criticising the guidance in a number of respects the judge laid down a number of controversial principles justifying his approach on the authority of the HRA.

1. A competent patient's decision as to his best interests and what treatment to receive or not was in principle determinative.
2. To withdraw treatment even where the patient was unaware could be a breach of Article 2 or 3.
3. The positive obligation of the State under articles 2 and 3 yielded to the patient's right to autonomy under Article 8.
4. A doctor unable or unwilling to carry out the wishes of a patient was under a duty to find another doctor who would. However, once the patient was in a coma there would be no breach of articles 2, 3, or 8 if artificial nutrition and hydration (ANH) was withdrawn where it was futile and served no purpose.
5. The obligations of a doctor and an NHS Trust could not be shed before they were taken over by someone else.
6. If the patient was incompetent the touchstone of best interests was intolerability and there was a strong presumption in favour of taking steps to prolong life.
7. Where there was doubt or disagreement as to a patient's competence, or as to whether ANH should be withdrawn, or where there was evidence that the patient if competent was resisting or disputing withdrawal of ANH, or where others with a claim to have their views taken into account asserted that withdrawal was contrary to the wishes of the patient or not in his bets interests, then in such cases there was a requirement to refer the case to court for a decision.
8. Although the Court might not make a mandatory order against a doctor to treat a patient, it could make a declaration, and could require a health authority to arrange for such treatment if to fail to do so would breach the patient's Convention rights.

The emphasis on the patient's wishes as to what treatment he should receive, not simply what treatment he should not, and the touchstone of the best interests of an incompetent patient being intolerability may subtly change the role of the doctor and the relationship between doctor and patient.

2. **Nearest Relative**
    (a) In *Re D* (Mental Patient: Habeas Corpus) (Nearest Relative) (2000) 2 FLR 848

The daughter of a patient who did not reside with him and had provided more than minimal care was consulted by an ASW as the nearest relative. The patient's detention was challenged as being unlawful on the grounds that his elder brother, rather than his daughter, was the nearest relative. The Court of Appeal held that:

(i) the correct question was whether the patient's daughter *appeared* to the ASW to be the nearest relative, not whether the ASW consulted with the nearest relative;

(ii) the word 'ordinarily' in Section 26(4) qualified 'resides with', but not 'is cared for' in the same section; and

(iii) there was no duty of reasonable enquiry on the part of the ASW as to who was the nearest relative.

Consequently, since the daughter had provided more than minimal care, but did not reside with the patient, the ASW was not wrong to consider her as the nearest relative.

(b) *R(S)* v. *City of Plymouth* (2002) 1 WLR 2583

The nearest relative of a patient lacking capacity applied for disclosure of the patient's (her daughter's) social services file so as to obtain advice as to whether an application (which she anticipated) to remove her as nearest relative under Section 29 of the Mental Health Act would be likely to succeed. The Local Authority refused on grounds of confidentiality, which they argued were not outweighed by other public interests. The mother failed before the High Court in her argument that this breached her rights under Article 6. She remained the patient's nearest relative with all the rights in respect of disclosure provided by the rules were an application to remove her under Section 29 in fact made. The matter went to the Court of Appeal by which time the Local Authority had altered its position so as to agree to disclosure of the information to the mother's experts but not directly to the mother or her solicitors. The Court of Appeal reversed the earlier decision and ordered disclosure to the mother and her solicitors. A balance had to be struck between the protection of confidentiality and the right of an interested party to information. In this case the balance came down in favour of disclosure. However, in so deciding the Court emphasized the importance of preserving confidentiality, including for the Learning Disabled, and where disclosure was given this should be strictly limited to reports which would have to be placed before the Court and should not be more widely circulated; the information to be disclosed would not include Social Services files.

(c) *R* v. *Liverpool City Council and Secretary of State for Health, ex parte SSG* (2002) 5 CCLR 639

First, in order in the statutory list to be the patient's nearest relative is his or her husband or wife. This includes heterosexual couples who have lived together as such for six months. However, same sex couples would have to live together for five years to qualify. This case held that this is discriminatory and contrary to the European Convention on Human Rights. In future same sex unmarried couples will only have to live together for six months to qualify.

(d) *R* v. *Secretary of State for Health, ex parte M* (2003) UKHRR 746; TLR 25/4/2003

It has long been a concern that the patient is not among those permitted to apply to the Court to replace his or her nearest relative. The patient may legitimately complain that the appointed nearest relative is an inappropriate person for many reasons, and indeed object to the implied breach of confidentiality that thereby occurs. That this is in breach of the patient's Convention rights was recognized some years ago in the case of *JT* v. *UK* when a 'friendly settlement' was reached before the European Court of Human Rights; the government gave an undertaking to amend the law. However, no amendment to Section 29 of the Mental Health Act has followed. The government plans to make changes in its proposed Mental Health Bill but these will not come into effect for several years. In this case the Court said that the delay was long enough and made a declaration under the Human Rights Act that Section 26 and Section 29 of the Mental Health Act were incompatible with the patient's rights under Article 8 of the European Convention. This, of course, does not of itself change the law which will still require parliament to make the necessary amendment. It remains to be seen whether the government acts under the fast-track procedure before any Mental Health Bill is introduced to parliament.

3. **Mental Health Review Tribunal Decisions**
   (a) *R v. Tower Hamlets Healthcare NHS Trust (MHRT, Discharge) Ex Parte Von Brandenburg* (2003) UKHL 58

The case concerns a patient detained under Section 2 whose Tribunal ordered his discharge, deferred for 7 days. Six days later the patient was detained on Section 3. It was submitted that there should have been at least a change of circumstances between the decision of the Tribunal and the renewed detention to justify such an action. At first instance the Court held that there was no such requirement for there to be a change of circumstances. This was in accordance with earlier case law which had, however, been criticized by a number of commentators. The Court of Appeal affirmed the decision that the fact that a Tribunal had ordered discharge was not a bar to a fresh application being made where the relevant health professionals believed that the criteria for detention existed. Such professionals are under a continuing duty to consider the appropriateness of these compulsory powers. However, the Court said that the circumstances would be rare in which a subsequent detention could be justified in the absence of a change of circumstances. The example was given of information coming to light subsequently which had not been available to the Tribunal. The professionals should not make a Section 3 application if they believe that another Tribunal would in fact order the patient's discharge following re-admission. While therefore the decision was upheld and the power of renewed detention confirmed, any such renewed detention would have to be taken after the most serious consideration of the Tribunal's decision.

The case has now reached the House of Lords, which has at last provided reasonably clear guidance on the powers and obligations of professionals faced with a Tribunal decision to discharge with which they disagree. The other Court of Appeal decision, noted at 3(e) below needs to be read in the light of this decision. In short the House of Lords confirmed:

(i) where a MHRT has ordered discharge of a patient it is lawful to re-admit him under Section 2 or Section 3 where it cannot be demonstrated that there has been a relevant change in circumstances. A conscientious doctor whose opinion has not been accepted by the Tribunal will ask whether his own opinion should be revised. But if he then adheres to his original opinion he cannot be obliged to suppress or alter it. His professional duty to his patient and his wider duty to the public require him to form, and if called upon express, the best professional judgement he can, whether or not that coincides with the judgement of the Tribunal.

(ii)   an ASW may not lawfully apply for the admission of a patient whose discharge has been ordered by the decision of a MHRT of which the ASW is aware unless the ASW has formed the reasonable and bona fide opinion that he has information not known to the Tribunal which puts a significantly different complexion on the case as compared with that which was before the Tribunal. Three examples were given:

1.   An ASW learns after a Tribunal decision that the patient made an earlier serious attempt on his life, not known to the Tribunal and which significantly alters the risk as assessed by the Tribunal.

2.   The Tribunal based a decision to discharge on the belief that the patient would take his medication (as he said he would). Before or after discharge he refuses to take his medication presenting a risk to himself or others.

3.   After the Tribunal decision the patient's mental condition significantly deteriorates so as to present a degree of risk or require treatment or supervision not evident at the hearing.

In such cases the ASW may properly apply for the admission of a patient, subject to the required medical support, notwithstanding a Tribunal decision to discharge.

(iii)   Although the 'relevant change of circumstances' test is not the correct one, the principle that tribunal decisions should be respected for what they decide means that if an ASW is making a fresh application to detain, the reasons for departing from the earlier decision should be given, albeit in general terms.

The alternative procedure (see 3(c) below) of not re-sectioning, but challenging the Tribunal decision while applying for a stay is probably only appropriate where what is in issue is whether the Tribunal has made a mistake in law.

(b) *R v. London South & South West Regional MHRT, Ex Parte Moyle* (2000) Lloyd's Rep 143

The applicant was subject to a Hospital Order and applied for discharge. Medical evidence showed that drugs controlled his illness and his condition was not such as would make it appropriate for him to be detained, but that if he were to stop taking his medication he would quickly relapse. The Tribunal was not satisfied that:

(i)   he would continue to take his medication if discharged; nor that

(ii)   his illness was not of a nature which made it appropriate for him to be detained.

Accordingly they rejected his application.

    The Court held that the criteria for discharge were meant to be matching or mirror images equivalent to the admission criteria. Whether a patient's illness made it appropriate for him to be detained depended upon an assessment of the probability that he might relapse. If a Tribunal was not satisfied that there was no probability of relapse in the near future it would be unlikely to be able to conclude that the criterion for continued detention had not been satisfied, because the nature if not the degree, of his disorder would warrant it. The refusal to discharge was remitted back to the Tribunal. This is an extension into English law of the principles developed in the

Scottish case of *Reid* v. *SOS* for Scotland. As a result of that case the issue of treatability, which formerly was not a consideration on discharge (the ruling in Canon's Park) has become a relevant factor in relation to Section 72. A Tribunal must find that it would be appropriate or necessary for a patient to be liable to be detained in the hospital for medical treatment prior to deciding to reject an application for discharge.

(c) *R (Ashworth SHA)* **v.** *MHRT W. Midlands and N.W. Region. R* **v.** *Oxfordshire MH Trust, ex parte H* (2002) EWCA Civ 923; TLR 10/7/2002

The case of *Brandenburg* (reported at 3(a) above), confirmed that a patient could lawfully be re-detained shortly after a Tribunal decision to discharge. The above two recent cases throw light on the circumstances in which in practice this can be done. In the Ashworth case a Tribunal peremptorily discharged a patient after hearing that no aftercare arrangements had been made for him. He was therefore re-detained under the Mental Health Act. This was challenged by the patient but at first instance the Court held that it was sufficient if the ASW and doctors were advised on substantial grounds, that the Tribunal's decision was unlawful and that proceedings to challenge it are at least imminent. They must act in accordance with their professional judgements and the patient's remedy is to apply to the Tribunal. The Tribunal should have adjourned for suitable aftercare provision to be arranged.

Thus to 'change in circumstances' or 'information not being available to the Tribunal' is added another example of where re-detention is lawful, even without a change in circumstances. However, this decision was reversed by the Court of Appeal which imposed tighter restrictions on re-sectioning in such circumstances:

(i)   Faced with such a situation the Hospital should have applied for Judicial Review of the Tribunal's decision, coupled with a stay which would act to 'turn the clock back' (unless perhaps the patient had already left).

(ii) The Healthcare professionals must ask themselves whether the main grounds for resectioning have effectively been rejected by the Tribunal.

(iii) An application to resection would need to be founded on circumstances unknown to the Tribunal.

In *ex parte H* the patient deteriorated in the period between the Tribunal's decision to discharge and the date fixed for discharge, and was re-detained. The patient's application for judicial review was refused. Although the professionals were bound to take into account the Tribunal's decision when making their application and recommendations this was not a case of differing professional views of the same circumstances but a deterioration outside the contemplation of the Tribunal at the time of ordering discharge.

The Brandenburg case (see 3(a) above) has reached the House of Lords and represents the current legal position. The suggestion that the correct procedure where there was disagreement with a Tribunal decision was to challenge it by judicial review coupled with an application for a stay is probably now best restricted to cases where the issue is whether the Tribunal has erred in law.

(d) *R* v. *Doncaster MBC, ex parte W* (2003) EWCA 192 Admin

This is another case, consistent with a line of recent cases concerning the extent of the obligation of the Health and Social Services Authorities to implement or comply with the conditions attached by a MHRT to its decision to discharge a detained patient. Here one of the conditions was that the patient should reside in appropriate accommodation approved by named doctors and social workers. This proved impossible to fulfil and so the patient remained detained. However, the MBC had used its best endeavours to find suitable accommodation and accordingly its duty under Section 117 had not been breached and there had been no unlawful detention.

The problem with this line of cases is that unless a Tribunal can enforce its decision (including conditions attaching to discharge) there is a potential breach of the patient's rights under Article 5(4) to be able effectively to challenge his detention. On the other hand, Courts have been reluctant to compel Authorities or clinicians to adopt a particular course which conflicts with their own reasonably held profession views. This issue was clarified when the case of *R(IH)* v. *Nottinghamshire Healthcare NHS Trust et al.* (2003) UKHL 59 went to the House of Lords.

(e) *R(IH)* v. *Nottinghamshire Healthcare NHS Trust* (2003) UKHL 59

In *R* v. *Camden and Islington Health Authority ex parte K* a patient remained detained because of the inability of the Authority to find a psychiatrist willing to supervise the patient in the community on the conditions set by the Tribunal. Section 117 did not impose an absolute requirement to satisfy the Tribunal's conditions and the resulting continued detention would not be in breach of Article 5. In *R(IH)* a similar impasse arose, and the issue was whether the lack of power in the Tribunal to enforce compliance with its conditions meant that there was a breach of the effective, speedy review provision of Article 5(4). The Court held that the Tribunal retained a monitoring role in such circumstances and that this power was sufficient to prevent a breach of Article 5(4). If the Tribunal did not exercise that power then there could be a breach of both Article 5(1)(e) and 5(4).

This decision was upheld by the Court of Appeal which set out some guidance on how such an impasse was to be resolved. It confirmed that a Tribunal *does* have the power to revisit its decision before a patient's discharge where conditions it has set have proved impossible to fulfil. It had been thought that the Tribunal lacked that power which gave rise to the argument that this would lead inevitably to a delay which might breach Article 5(4) by leaving the patient in limbo.

The case has now been heard by the House of Lords which confirmed that the obligation in respect of conditions for discharge of a restricted patient set by a Tribunal is to use best endeavours, rather than absolute. A failure to use best endeavours or to act in good faith could lead to challenge. The fact that a Tribunal lacked the power to secure compliance with its conditions did not mean it lacked the necessary attributes of a court as required by Article 5(4). The Court of Appeal's new guidance was correct, from which it followed that Tribunals should reconsider conditions which turned out to be impracticable and if this led to the continued detention of the patient that would not be unlawful. The individual professional autonomy of the consultant psychiatrist has therefore been preserved. The House of Lords left open whether a Community RMO was a hybrid Public Authority and thus covered by the requirement of the HRA not to act in a way incompatible with an individual's Convention rights.

(f) R v. MHRT, ex parte Li [2004] EWHC 51 Admin

In the light of the House of Lords decision in *Von Brandenburg* (see 3(a) above) this case assumes greater importance as the Approved Social Worker, when deciding whether to make a fresh application to detain a patient will clearly need to know the basis of and reasons for the Tribunal's decision to discharge in sufficient detail to be able to decide if fresh information would be likely to have put a significantly different complexion on the case. The present case involved a successful application to judicially review a Tribunal's decision on the basis that the reasons given were inadequate. Fuller decisions are likely to be required in future, and quickly enough for an ASW to respond appropriately in cases falling within Von Brandenburg criteria.

4.   **Miscellaneous Cases**

(a) Re F (A Child) (2000) 1 FLR 192

The Court of Appeal held that the definition of mental impairment associated with seriously irresponsible conduct in Section 1(2) of the Mental Health Act 1983 should be given a restrictive construction and in so holding the Court allowed a father's appeal against the Guardianship Order in respect of his daughter. The Judge had originally held that F suffered from mental impairment and that her desire to return home from the specialist children's home, constituted 'seriously irresponsible conduct'. The importance of this case is that it emphasizes the difficulty placed in the way of Local Authorities and others in utilizing Guardianship Orders in cases which might otherwise be thought to be appropriate. Take, for instance, the renowned Beverley Lewis Inquest where a severely mentally impaired woman lived with her mentally ill mother and did not receive the care that she needed, subsequently dying. Because Beverley Lewis was passive, and her disability not associated with abnormally aggressive or seriously irresponsible conduct, a Guardianship Order could not be obtained even though that might have best met her needs in the circumstances. A revision of the criteria for guardianship still requires reconsideration.

(b) Re F (Adult Patient: Jurisdiction) (2000) 3 WLR 1740

A different point concerning the same patient came before the Court of Appeal again in June 2000. F had now reached the age of 18 and the question arose whether the Local Authority could apply for declarations that it would continue both to require that she remain in local authority accommodation and to restrict access on the part of her family.

The Local Authority decided that such declarations could be made, following the Bournewood decision, on grounds of necessity which was not limited to medical and similar short-term emergencies, nor to the statutory guardianship or other provisions of the Mental Health Act. Nor did this breach Article 5 of the European Convention because it was a procedure prescribed by law, as was the requirement, and would not be overridden by any regard for the right to family life of F's mother or other relatives under Article 8.

(c) Epsom & St Helier NHS Trust v. MHRT(W) (2001) EWCA Admin 101

This case throws further light on the question what degree of continuing inpatient treatment is required to justify renewing a patient's Section 3 detention while the patient is on Section 17 leave. Since the decision in *Re Barker* it has been possible, provided that there is such an element of in-patient treatment, to renew a patient's detention while on leave, a situation which was previously regarded as having been outlawed by the case of *R* v. *Hallstrom*. In the Epsom case the patient was on leave of absence to a nursing home which was not a registered mental nursing home. While *Re Barker* clarified the law, it did not define the degree of inpatient treatment that would be required. In the Epsom case there was no current inpatient treatment, simply the prospect or likelihood of treatment being required in the future during the period of detention under Section 3. That was held by the Court to be insufficient.

(d) *R (DR)* v. *Mersey Care NHS Trust* TLR 11/10/2002

Unlike in the Epsom & St Helier case above, while the correct test for renewal of detention was whether the criteria set by Section 20(4)(a) and Section 3(2)(a) had been met (whether the plan for the patient was for her to receive medical treatment in hospital), in this case of a 'revolving door' patient a significant component in the care plan was for treatment in hospital. The test was satisfied and the fact that the plan also included extended leave of absence did not invalidate the detention.

(e) *Reed (Trainer)* v. *Bronglais Hospital etc.* (2001) EWHC Admin 792

One of the two medical recommendations required to support an application for admission under Section 2 of the Mental Health Act must, if practicable by Section 12(2), be from a practitioner who has previous acquaintance with the patient. In this case the issue before the Court was what constituted 'previous acquaintance'. Here the doctor in question:

(i)   attended a case conference which gave much background information on the patient and included the minutes of two previous case conferences

(ii)   following the case conference, saw the patient for about 5 minutes

(iii) 'scanned' the medical records received from the Family Health Authority (sic)

(iv)   then saw the patient again to make his recommendation.

The Court held that the words should be given their ordinary meaning and that the reference in the Code of Practice to 'personal' knowledge did not import any greater requirement. The doctor had sufficient 'previous acquaintance', and any doctor would have who had some previous knowledge of the patient and was not coming to him or her 'cold'.

(f) *Keenan* v. *UK* Hudoc 27229/95

Although the threshold for a breach of Article 3 of the European Convention is high, the Convention is a dynamic instrument which should be interpreted in the light of changing social attitudes and medical advances. There is the suggestion therefore that as a result the threshold might gradually be lowered. Support for this view is to be found in the recent case of *Keenan* v. *UK*. Mr Keenan died in prison by hanging himself. He had longstanding psychiatric illness. The Court found that the lack of effective monitoring of his condition in prison and the lack of informed psychiatric input into his assessment and treatment disclosed significant defects in the medical care provided to a mentally ill person known to be a suicide risk. To add to this he sustained a serious disciplinary punishment including segregation. This was held to be incompatible with the standard of treatment required in respect of a mentally ill person and as such breached Article 3. The comment by the Court that the lack of appropriate medical treatment could amount to treatment contrary to Article 3 is highly significant, as was the comment that in the case of mentally ill persons their vulnerability had to be taken into consideration in terms of how they might be affected by treatment, or the lack of it, or punishment.

(g) *S v. Airedale NHS Trust et al.* (2002) EWHC 1780 Admin
**   *Munjaz v. Mersey Care NHS Trust* (2003) EWCA Civ 1036**

The Court of Appeal has now considered the legality of seclusion in these two cases in the context of the domestic private law, the European Convention, and the Code of Practice. The principles emerging from this judgement are:

(i)   At Common Law seclusion might be justified for informal patients on the basis of what was reasonably necessary to protect the patient and others from immediate risk of harm.

(ii)   Seclusion could constitute 'medical treatment' for the purposes of Section 63 of the Mental Health Act, but the principle of 'reasonable necessity' applied.

(iii) In some circumstances the use of seclusion might involve a tort for which the patient could sue (e.g. use of excessive force) but not the use of seclusion per se, even if it did not comply with the Code of Practice.

(iv)   Article 5 was not concerned with the conditions of detention but with whether the detention was lawful.

(v)   Article 3 might be breached if the conditions of detention defeated rather than promoted the assessment and treatment of the patient's mental disorder.

(vi)   Seclusion was caught by Article 8(1) but could be justified under Article 8(2). The Code of Practice was relevant in determining whether any breach was justified.

(vii) The Code of Practice should be followed by all hospitals unless they have a good reason for departing from it in relation to an individual patient. They may identify good reasons for particular departures in relation to groups of patients who share particular well defined characteristics, but they cannot depart from it as a matter of policy.

(viii) Although the Court of Appeal's comments concerning the applicability of the Code of Practice referred specifically to the issue of seclusion, they are likely to be relevant to other practice areas.

Section	Purpose	Maximum duration	Can patient apply to MHRT?	Can nearest relative apply to MHRT?	Will there be an automatic MHRT hearing?	Do consent-to-treatment rules apply?*
2	Admission for assessment	28 days; not renewable	Within first 14 days	No: Section 23 gives them power to discharge, but see Section 25 below	No	Yes
3	Admission for treatment	6 months; may be renewed for 6 months and then yearly	Within first 6 months and then in each period	No: Section 23 gives them power to discharge, but see Section 25 below	If one has not been held, managers refer to MHRT at 6 months and then every 3 years (annually if patient is under age 16 years)	Yes
4	Admission for assessment in an emergency	72 h; not renewable, but second doctor can change to Section 2	Yes, but only relevant if Section 4 is converted to a Section 2	No	No	No
5(2)	Doctor's holding power	72 h; not renewable	No	No	No	No
5(4)	Nurse's holding power	6 h; not renewable, but doctor can change to Section 5(2)	No	No	No	No
7	Reception into guardianship	6 months; may be renewed for 6 months and then yearly	Within first 6 months and then in each period	No: Section 23 gives them power to discharge	No	No
16	Doctor reclassifies the mental disorder	For the duration of the detention	Within 28 days of being informed	Within 28 days of being informed	No	–
19	Transfer from guardianship to hospital	6 months; may be renewed for 6 months and then yearly	In the first 6 months of detention and then in each period	No: Section 23 gives them power to discharge, but see Section 25 below	If one has not been held, managers refer to MHRT at 6 months and then every 3 years (annually if patient is under age 16 years)	Yes

ii Summary of civil treatment codes

Section	Purpose	Maximum duration	Can patient apply to MHRT?	Can nearest relative apply to MHRT?	Will there be an automatic MHRT hearing?	Do consent-to-treatment rules apply?*
25	Restriction of discharge by nearest relative	Variable	No	Within 28 days of being informed (no appeal if Section 2)	No	–
25A	Supervised aftercare	6 months; may be renewed for 6 months and then yearly	Within first 6 months and then in each period	Yes, if entitled to be informed, once in each period	No	No
29	Appointment of acting nearest relative by court	Variable	No	Within 1 year and then yearly	No	–
135	Warrant to search for and remove patient	72 h; not renewable	No	No	No	No
136	Police power in public places	72 h; not renewable	No	No	No	No

MHRT, Mental Health Review Tribunal.
*Where consent-to-treatment rules do not apply, the patient is in the same position as an informal patient and should not be treated without his or her consent, except in an emergency under common law.

Under Section 67, the Secretary of State can refer Part II patients to the MHRT at any time.

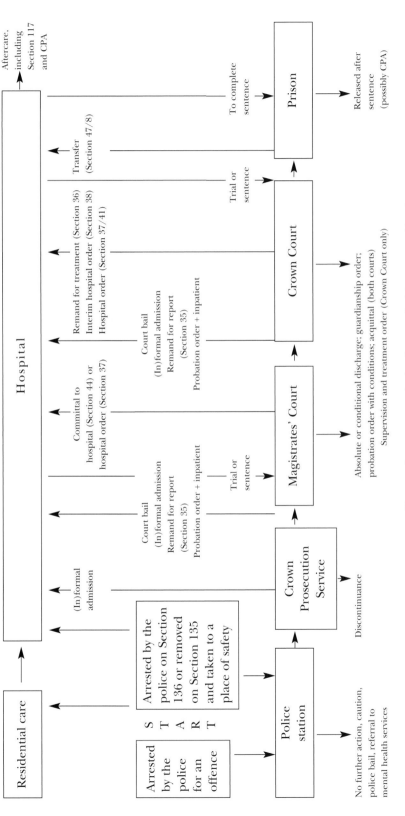

111 The police, the courts and public health

All section references are from the Mental Health Act 1983.

IV Flowchart of decisions involving consent to treatment

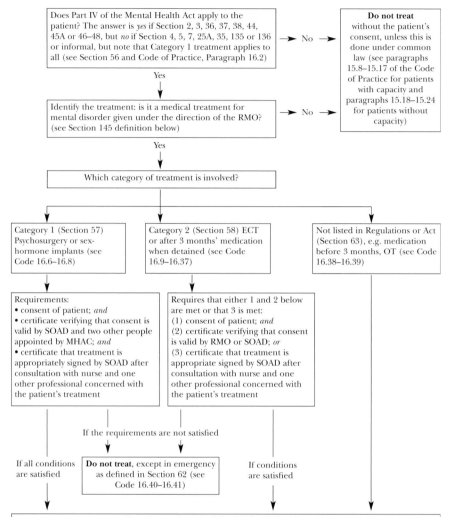

Does Part IV of the Mental Health Act apply to the patient? The answer is *yes* if Section 2, 3, 36, 37, 38, 44, 45A or 46–48, but *no* if Section 4, 5, 7, 25A, 35, 135 or 136 or informal, but note that Category 1 treatment applies to all (see Section 56 and Code of Practice, Paragraph 16.2)

→ No →

Do not treat without the patient's consent, unless this is done under common law (see paragraphs 15.8–15.17 of the Code of Practice for patients with capacity and paragraphs 15.18–15.24 for patients without capacity)

Yes ↓

Identify the treatment: is it a medical treatment for mental disorder given under the direction of the RMO? (see Section 145 definition below)

→ No →

Yes ↓

Which category of treatment is involved?

Category 1 (Section 57) Psychosurgery or sex-hormone implants (see Code 16.6–16.8)

Category 2 (Section 58) ECT or after 3 months' medication when detained (see Code 16.9–16.37)

Not listed in Regulations or Act (Section 63), e.g. medication before 3 months, OT (see Code 16.38–16.39)

Requirements:
• consent of patient; *and*
• certificate verifying that consent is valid by SOAD and two other people appointed by MHAC; *and*
• certificate that treatment is appropriately signed by SOAD after consultation with nurse and one other professional concerned with the patient's treatment

Requires that either 1 and 2 below are met or that 3 is met:
(1) consent of patient; *and*
(2) certificate verifying that consent is valid by RMO or SOAD; *or*
(3) certificate that treatment is appropriate signed by SOAD after consultation with nurse and one other professional concerned with the patient's treatment

If the requirements are not satisfied

If all conditions are satisfied

Do not treat, except in emergency as defined in Section 62 (see Code 16.40–16.41)

If conditions are satisfied

Treat, but see Paragraph 16.4 of the Code of Practice
'A detained patient is not necessarily incapable of giving consent. The patient's consent should be sought for all proposed treatments which may lawfully be given under the Act. It is the personal responsibility of the patient's current RMO to ensure that valid consent has been sought. The interview at which such consent was sought should be properly recorded in the medical notes.'

ECT, electroconvulsive therapy; MHAC, Mental Health Act Commission; OT, occupational therapy; RMO, responsible medical officer; SOAD, second-opinion appointed doctor.
'Medical treatment' is defined in Section 145 as including 'nursing, and also includes care, habilitation and rehabilitation under medical supervision' (see also Code, Paragraph 15.4).

Form 2

Application by an approved social worker for admission for assessment

Mental Health Act 1983
Section 2

To the Managers of

(name and address of hospital or mental nursing home)

ROYAL WESSEX HOSPITAL, WESSEX NHS PARTNERSHIP TRUST
HIPARDI AVENUE, CASTERBRIDGE,
WESSEX, GG20 1RU

(your full name)

I MALCOLM PRACTICE

(your office address)

of ANGST HOUSE, DECISION STREET, CASTERBRIDGE GG12PT

hereby apply for the admission of

(full name of patient)

AGATHA ROYAL

(address of patient)

of 24 HARDY AVENUE
CASTERBRIDGE, WESSEX, GG17 2BU

for assessment in accordance with Part II of the Mental Health Act 1983.

(name of local social services authority)

I am an officer of WESSEX COUNTY COUNCIL

appointed to act as an approved social worker for the purposes of the Act.

Indicate clearly below if the nearest relative is known or not.

The following section should be completed if nearest relative known.

Indicate if (a) or (b) is applicable

(a) To the best of my knowledge and belief

(name and address)

DEBORAH ROYAL
2 CACKLE ROW, BANK ST. JOHN,
CASTERBRIDGE, GG42 6RU

is the patient's nearest relative within the meaning of the Act.

delete the phrase which does not apply

I have
~~I have not yet~~

informed that person that this application is to be made and of his power to order the discharge of the patient.

OR

(b) I understand that

(name and address)

has been authorised by

delete the phrase which does not apply

a county court
the patient's nearest relative.

Please turn over

to exercise the functions under the Act of the patient's nearest relative.

delete the phrase which
does not apply

I have
I have not yet

informed that person that this application is to be made and of his power to order the discharge of the patient.

*The following section should be completed **if nearest relative not known***

delete the phrase
which does not
apply

(a) I have been unable to ascertain who is this patient's nearest relative within the meaning of the Act.

OR

(b) To the best of my knowledge and belief this patient has no nearest relative within the meaning of the Act.

The following section must be completed in all cases

(date) I last saw the patient on

20ᵗʰ JULY 2004

I have interviewed the patient and I am satisfied that detention in a hospital is in all the circumstances of the case the most appropriate way of providing the care and medical treatment of which the patient stands in need.

This application is founded on two medical recommendations in the prescribed form.

If neither of the medical practitioners knew the patient before making their recommendations, please explain why you could not get a recommendation from a medical practitioner who did know the patient:-

This is a first presentation with a mental disorder and I have not been able to find a GP who knows Agatha Royal.

Signed _Malcolm Partin_   Date _20/07/04_

Form 4

Mental Health Act 1983
Section 2

Medical recommendation for admission for assessment

(full name and address of medical practitioner)

I   BARBARA INA SOCK

ROYAL WESSEX HOSPITAL, HIPARDI AVENUE
CASTERBRIDGE, WESSEX GG20 1RU

a registered medical practitioner, recommend that

(full name and address of patient)

AGATHA ROYAL

24 HARDY AVENUE
CASTERBRIDGE, WESSEX, GG17 2BU

be admitted to a hospital for assessment in accordance with Part II of the Mental Health Act 1983.

I last examined this patient on

(date)   20th JULY 2004

*Delete if not applicable

*I had previous acquaintance with the patient before I conducted that examination.

*I have been approved by the Secretary of State under section 12 of the Act as having special experience in the diagnosis or treatment of mental disorder.

I am of the opinion

(a) that this patient is suffering from mental disorder of a nature or degree which warrants detention of the patient in a hospital for assessment

AND

Delete the indents not applicable

(b) that this patient ought to be so detained
   (i) in the interests of the patient's own health
   (ii) in the interests of patient's own safety
   (iii) with a view to the protection of other persons

AND

(c) that informal admission is not appropriate in the circumstances of this case for the following reasons:-

(The full reasons why informal admission is not appropriate must be given)

The patient is refusing the offer of a bed and will not co-operate with any treatment plan as she says there is nothing wrong.

Signed _____   Date 20th Jly 2004

Printed in the U.K. for H.M.S.O. 8476477 3/96 36K 67067

Form 9
Application by approved social worker
for admission for treatment

Mental Health Act 1983
Section 3

To the Managers of

(name and address
of hospital or
mental nursing home)

> ROYAL WESSEX HOSPITAL, WESSEX NHS PARTNERSHIP TRUST
> HIPARDI AVENUE, CASTERBRIDGE
> WESSEX, GG20 IRU

(your full name) I

> MALCOLM PRACTICE

(your office address) of

> ANGST HOUSE, DECISION STREET,
> CASTERBRIDGE, WESSEX, GG12FT

hereby apply for the admission of

(full name of patient)

> AGATHA ROYAL

(address of patient) of

> 24 HARDY AVENUE
> CASTERBRIDGE, WESSEX, GG17 2BU

for treatment in accordance with Part II of the Mental Health Act 1983 as a person suffering from:

mental illness, mental impairment, severe mental impairment, psychopathic disorder

(enter whichever
of these is
appropriate)

> MENTAL ILLNESS

I am an officer of

(name of local social
services authority)

> WESSEX COUNTY COUNCIL

appointed to act as an approved social worker for the purposes of the Act.

Indicate clearly below if the nearest relative has been consulted or not.

The following section should be completed where consultation has taken place

Complete (a) or (b)

(name and address)   (a) I have consulted

> DEBORAH ROYAL
> 2 CACKLE ROW, BANK ST. JOHN
> CASTERBRIDGE, GG42 6RU

who to the best of my knowledge and belief is the patient's nearest relative within the meaning of the Act

That person known as the nearest relative has not notified me or the local social services authority by whom I am appointed that he/she objects to this application being made.

Please turn over

OR

(name and address)   (b) I have consulted

who I understand has been authorised by

Delete the phrase   a county court
which does not
apply   the patient's nearest relative

to exercise the functions under the Act of the patient's nearest relative.

That person known as the nearest relative has not notified me or the local social services authority by whom I am appointed that he/she objects to this application being made.

The following section should be completed where <u>no</u> consultation has taken place.

Indicate whether   (a) I have been unable to ascertain who is this patient's nearest relative within the meaning
(a) (b) or (c) applies   of the Act.

OR

(b) To the best of my knowledge and belief this patient has no nearest relative within the meaning of the Act.

OR

(name and address)   (c) I understand that

is

delete either   (i) this patient's nearest relative within the meaning of the Act
(i) or (ii)   (ii) authorised to exercise the functions of this patient's nearest relative under the Act

AND in my opinion it is not reasonably practicable or would involve unreasonable delay to consult that person before making this application

The following section must be completed in all cases

(date)   I last saw the patient on   10th AUGUST 2004

! have interviewed the patient and I am satisfied that detention in a hospital is in all the circumstances of the case the most appropriate way of providing the care and medical treatment of which the patient stands in need.

The application is founded on two medical recommendations in the prescribed form.

Continued

If neither of the medical practitioners knew the patient before making their recommendations, please explain why you could not get a recommendation from a medical practitioner who did know the patient:-

_____

_____

_____

_____

_____

_____

Signed _____ Date _____ 10/08/08

Form 11

Medical recommendation for admission for treatment

Mental Health Act 1983
Section 3

(full name and address of practitioner)

I

BARBARA INA SOCK

ROYAL WESSEX HOSPITAL, HIPARDI AVENUE

CASTERBRIDGE, WESSEX, GG20 IRU

a registered medical practitioner, recommend that

(full name and address of patient)

AGATHA ROYAL

24 HARDY AVENUE

CASTERBRIDGE, WESSEX, GG17 2BU

be admitted to hospital for treatment in accordance with Part II of the Mental Health Act 1983.

(date) I last examined this patient on

10u AUGUST 2004

*Delete if not applicable

*(a) I had previous acquaintance with the patient before I conducted that examination.

*(b) I have been approved by the Secretary of State under section 12 of the Act as having special experience in the diagnosis or treatment of mental disorder.

In my opinion this patient is suffering from —

(complete (a) or (b))

(a) mental illness/~~severe mental impairment~~ **and his mental disorder is of a nature or degree which makes it appropriate for him to receive medical treatment in a hospital;

**The phrase which does not apply must be deleted

(b) ~~psychopathic disorder/mental impairment~~ **and ~~his mental disorder is of a nature or, degree which makes it appropriate for him to receive medical treatment in a hospital and such treatment is likely to alleviate or prevent a deterioration of his condition.~~

This opinion is founded on the following grounds:-
[Give clinical description of the patient's mental condition]

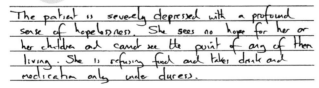

The patient is severely depressed with a profound sense of hopelessness. She sees no hope for her or her children and cannot see the point of any of them living. She is refusing food and takes drink and medication only under duress.

I am of the opinion that it is necessary

Delete the indents not applicable

(i) in the interest of the patient's own health
(ii) in the interest of patient's own safety
(iii) with a view to the protection of other persons

Please turn over

that this patient should receive treatment and it cannot be provided unless he is detained under section 3 of the Act, for the following reasons:-

[Reasons should indicate whether other methods of care or treatment (eg out-patient treatment or local social services authority services) are available and if so why they are not appropriate, and why informal admission is not appropriate.]

She is refusing food and would leave the hospital if she could. Only takes medication because she has been told she must do so.

Signed _____ Bab Such _____ Date 10/08/04

Subject Index

Notes

Legal cases are cited as presented in the text, and cross-references from the second name (defendant) are assumed.
Page numbers followed by 'f' indicate figures; page numbers followed by 't' indicate tables.

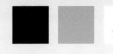